PATIENT ACCOUNT MANAGEMENT

Allen G. Herkimer, Jr.

Assistant Professor
California State University
Northridge

Principal
Alfa Management Services

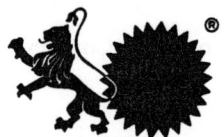

AN ASPEN PUBLICATION®
Aspen Systems Corporation
Rockville, Maryland
London
1983

Library of Congress Cataloging in Publication Data

Herkimer, Allen G.
Patient account management.

Includes bibliographies and index.
1. Hospitals—Accounting. I. Title. [DNLM:
1. Accounting—Methods. 2. Economics, Hospital.
WX 157 H548p]
HF5686.H7H4 1983 657'.8322 82-16318
ISBN: 0-89443-835-2

Publisher: John Marozsan
Editorial Director: Michael Brown
Managing Editor: Margot Raphael
Editorial Services: Eileen Higgins
Printing and Manufacturing: Debbie Collins

Copyright © 1983 by Aspen Systems Corporation

All rights reserved. This book, or parts thereof, may not be reproduced in any form or by any means, electronic or mechanical, including photocopy, recording, or any information storage and retrieval system now known or to be invented, without written permission from the publisher, except in the case of brief quotations embodied in critical articles or reviews. For information, address Aspen Systems Corporation, 1600 Research Boulevard, Rockville, Maryland 20850.

Library of Congress Catalog Card Number: 82-16318
ISBN: 0-89443-835-2

Printed in the United States of America

1 2 3 4 5

*To the patient account managers I've known
and to those I have yet to meet*

Table of Contents

Foreword ix

Preface xi

Acknowledgments xiii

Chapter 1— Organizing the Patient Business Services Department   1

    Role of the Patient Account Manager 1
    Department Mission 3
    Missions Defined 4
    Management Planning Defined 6
    Organizational Design 6
    Delegation of Authority 14
    Job Analysis 15
    Job Description 16
    Summary 17

Chapter 2— The Use of Standard Plans 21

    Policies 21
    Procedures 22
    Methods 25
    Benefits of Standard Plans 25

Chapter 3— The Hospital Accounting Process 27

    Double Entry Bookkeeping 28
    Accrual Accounting 30
    Fund Accounting 33

Prerequisites of an Accounting System 34
The Accounting Process 39
Application of the Accounting Process 48

Chapter 4— Management Accounting and Its Application **59**
Management Reporting 60
Principles of Expense Behavior 62
Other Expense Classifications 69
Cost Analysis 70
Application of Expense Behavior Principles 73
Variance Analysis 80

Chapter 5— Developing a Productivity Improvement Program **89**
Production Unit 90
Selection of Production Units 92
Staffing and Budgetary Control 94
Evaluating Departmental Performance 98
Employee Performance Evaluation 101
Employee Incentive Plans 104
Cost Allocation 107
Development of Production Standards 108

Chapter 6— The Budgetary Control System **117**
Role of the Patient Account Manager 120
Functional and Responsibility Budgeting 120
Types of Budgets 124
The Budgetary Control System 125

Chapter 7— Application of Variable Budgeting **133**
Purpose of Variable Budgeting 133
Relationship of Standard Costs to Variable Budgeting 134
Developing Standard Rates and Costs 135
Developing the Variable Budget 136
Developing the Direct-Variable Control Budget 145
Analysis of Salary Budget Variances 147
Analysis of Nonsalary Expense Variances 152
Step-Variable Staffing and Variance Analysis 157

Chapter 8— The Cost Finding Process **163**
Methods of Cost Finding 165

Table of Contents vii

        Keys to the Cost Finding Process 166
        A Cost Finding Case Study 169

Chapter 9— Financial Requirements and Rate Setting **179**

        Financial Requirements 180
        Third Party Impact on Published Rates 181
        Case Study of Reimbursement Procedures 182
        Rate Setting 190

Chapter 10—Cash Forecasting and Management **195**

        Purpose 195
        Major Components 196
        Cash Forecasting Methodology 201
        Role of the Patient Account Manager 215

Chapter 11—Analyzing the Financial Statements **219**

        Use of Financial Ratios 219
        Types of Ratio Analysis 222
        Liquidity of Patient Accounts Receivable 237
        Another Look at Financial Statements 241

Chapter 12—Payment and Collection for Services Rendered **245**

        Published Charge Versus Payment 247
        Classification of Payers 248
        Payment Systems 248
        Segmentation of Patient Accounts Receivable 249
        Monitoring Accounts in Collection 250
        Other Methods of Improving Payment 253

Chapter 13—Internal Audit and Control of Receivables **255**

        Internal Audit 256
        Internal Control 257
        Financial Versus Operational Auditing 258
        External Versus Internal Auditing 259
        Patient Business Services Audit Instrument 261
        Flow Charting 261
        Role of the Patient Account Manager 278

Foreword

Allen Herkimer has accomplished two giant steps in authoring this book.

First, he has recognized the specialized field of patient account management and is a prime force in increasing professionalization in this field.

The medical profession long ago realized the need for lay people to administer their health care facilities and created the position of hospital administrator. As the field became more technical and complex, sophisticated knowledge and training were required and, in the 1930s, the need for professional hospital administrators was recognized. Because of the increased diversity of operational skills required of the administrator, financial recordkeeping functions were turned over to the bookkeeper. Again, increasing financial complexity and sophistication required a more highly trained, skilled, and creative person and, in the 1950s, this group professionalized as financial officers and financial managers. They, in turn, delegated reimbursement and cash flow problems to credit managers because of another explosion in the fields of reimbursement, cash flow, management, patient relations, and collection activity. These skills are discussed in this book. They now require a highly educated, technically sophisticated individual. As a result, the profession of patient account management is now in the embryonic stage of development. Allen Herkimer's experience and sensitivity in the field of health care management resulted in his being one of the first to recognize this development.

As a result, the author has accomplished the second giant step, which is to define the knowledge, information, and skills required by the professional manager of patient accounts. This book is important not only because it sets forth the definition, but because it also educates the reader with the management, economic, and financial information needed to be a professional. To my knowledge, this is the first time that this subject matter has been presented in a single source for the manager of patient accounts.

Allan M. Tabas, Esq.
December 1982

Preface

During the past decade a silent but steady evolution has been taking place in the health care industry, especially within hospitals.

A decade ago the individual who was in charge of handling and collecting the hospital's receivables was commonly called a credit manager. Even the title was a misnomer because this individual did not grant credit. The hospital Board of Directors handled this particular function.

By stating that no person entering the facility would be refused patient care, this well meaning group of community minded persons opened the doors: credit granting had been mandated.

The credit manager's role was threefold:

1. to establish some type of payoff procedure, whether it was total cash collection at discharge or through some method of systematic amortization of the patient's debt
2. to establish and conduct a routine billing and follow-up procedure for unpaid accounts
3. to refer uncollectible accounts to professional collection agencies

That was only ten years ago.

Since then the credit manager's job description, role, and title have changed. The position has gained recognition and has achieved importance on the hospital's management team. This increase in "status" is due primarily to less philanthropic donations and public grants; the hospital has been forced to depend almost entirely on its own operations for needed cash. The former hospital credit manager now answers to a variety of titles, among them:

- patient account manager
- business office manager

- assistant controller
- director of patient business services
- vice president—patient economic relations

Most important, along with the title changes, the areas of responsibility and authority that go with the position have also changed. Today's patient account manager is expected to:

- recommend patient business service policies and to manage and implement these policies
- know third party reimbursement systems and assist with developing methods to maximize cash receipts
- develop, organize, and manage appropriate admitting, discharge, billing, and collection procedures within the approved hospital policies
- contribute to the design of a data processing system that will expedite the analysis and collection of accounts receivable
- assist in rate setting
- assist in cash flow projections and management
- develop and monitor employee performance standards
- assist in various routine accounting procedures
- develop a management information system that will identify weaknesses in departmental responsibility areas
- coordinate procedures; manage and evaluate people
- act as a "salesperson" for the hospital

Over the past several years, I have received letters and/or comments from participants at seminars I've conducted telling me that there is a need for a book written especially for the patient account manager. Such a book, I've been told, should include the previously mentioned responsibility areas but should emphasize the technical skills needed for the position in today's hospital environment.

In response to their stated need, this book has been written; it is dedicated to those individuals who have experienced the evolution of the credit manager and who have contributed to the growth and development of the *new* professional in this position.

The book is designed for the modern receivables manager, for the person who has responsibility for maintaining a favorable hospital image and good public relations while bringing in the cash.

Allen G. Herkimer Jr., M.B.A., F.H.F.M.A., C.M.P.A.
December 1982

Acknowledgments

Samuel Johnson stated that "Nobody can write the life of a man but those who have eat and drunk and lived in social intercourse with him."* Accordingly, this book could never have been written if I had not actually worked and socialized with patient account managers and other health care professionals too numerous to identify and to count. To these people, I owe a considerable amount of gratitude. I have assimilated much knowledge from these individuals and recognized some of the management tools required to effectively and efficiently administer the patient business services department.

However, the following are key individuals who were directly involved in developing and writing this book:

First, Robert Rolfsen and my wife, Fay, planted the seed to develop a "get-acquainted" hospital accounting book especially for the patient account manager.

Second, I am grateful to Patricia Rummer for assisting in the initial editing of the book; her knowledge and experience in editing in the field of patient account management were invaluable.

Finally, I wish to acknowledge the patient account managers of the future in whose hands we have placed the viability of this nation's hospital industry.

---

* John Bartlett, *Familiar Quotations* (Boston, Mass.: Little, Brown & Co., 1952), p. 235.

Chapter 1

Organizing the Patient Business Services Department

ROLE OF THE PATIENT ACCOUNT MANAGER

The most important role of the patient account manager is to manage the department effectively—to mobilize and manipulate its human and material resources efficiently so that the department reaches its established goals and objectives. Most economic and social goals are reached through organized group effort; managing the patient account department, then, can be the key to meeting the hospital's financial and social responsibilities.

Management has been defined as the creation and maintenance of an internal environment in which individuals, working together in groups, can perform efficiently and effectively toward the attainment of group goals. Managing is, in fact, the art of doing, and management is the body of organized knowledge that underlies the art.[1]

This definition includes the following key words:

- creation
- internal environment
- working together
- efficiently
- effectively
- goals

The patient account manager must create an environment that enhances working conditions and improves productivity. It must be the kind of environment within which dissension and inefficiency are minimized while productivity and high employee morale are maximized. The patient account manager, with the cooperation of the department supervisors, is responsible for maintaining these working conditions within the internal environment. This kind of team attitude must not be limited to intradepartmental activities but must extend to other departments and be exhibited attitudinally throughout the hospital.

There are two important points to remember about being an effective manager:

1. The department manager establishes the mode and/or style of management and the department's working climate.
2. The manager must select a management style that is comfortable and workable for him or her.

Traditionally, most management styles are based on Douglas McGregor's "Theory X" and "Theory Y" or some combination of the two. According to McGregor:

- A "Theory X" manager assumes that people are fundamentally lazy, irresponsible, and need constantly to be watched.
- A "Theory Y" manager assumes that people are fundamentally hardworking, responsible, and need only to be supported and encouraged.[2]

One more management theory has recently come into focus. Japan's "Theory Z" suggests that when an important decision needs to be made, everyone who will feel its impact must be involved in making it; that is, the worker is also a planner and engineer. "Theory Z" assumes that:

- More important than the decision itself is people's commitment.
- Everyone must be well informed about the decision to be made.[3]

Whichever management style he or she selects, the patient account manager must keep the primary goal always in focus—to maintain the working capital required to finance the hospital's accounts receivable at a realistic minimum. The effective management of patient accounts receivable is the single most important factor in the financial success of a hospital. An efficient patient account function can literally prevent bankruptcy.

Effective management of patient accounts receivable involves more than just collecting money. The patient account department performs many other functions, including:

- establishing a charge structure for patient services that appropriately covers the hospital's total financial requirements
- designing accounting and cost allocation systems and procedures that maximize reimbursement

- maintaining open communication with third party reimbursement (payment) agencies in order to improve the hospital's financial position
- assuring that the medical records and social services functions are adequately performed so that timely billing and patient referral is possible
- maintaining cooperation and communication with medical staff to assure timely completion of patient charts and adequate patient information
- developing appropriate performance standards and adhering to them

These functions are the responsibility of the patient account manager, and they make his or her job much more complex than it was 15 years ago. Among other responsibilities, today's patient account manager is expected to perform the functions of the following:

- systems analyst
- systems designer
- personnel manager
- public relations representative
- reimbursement negotiator
- collection agent
- policy and procedure analyst

Data processing, for example, is one function which increasingly demands the patient account manager's time. Whether the data processing system is manual or electronic, effective performance of this function is a major key to the manager's success, as well as that of his or her department and the entire hospital. The hospital administrator may assign other functions to the patient account manager depending on the hospital's needs, the area of responsibility in which the patient account management function is placed, and the manager's abilities; but the need for timely, accurate, and meaningful information is always present.

DEPARTMENT MISSION

The health care industry is dynamic, and the patient account manager's position is no less dynamic. Today's patient account managers must be trailblazers in carrying out this ever-challenging hospital administrative position. In order to succeed, they must establish a formal mission or purpose for the department.

Whether the patient account managers select a traditional organizational structure for the department, choose the patient service representative system, or opt for a combination of the two approaches, they must adopt and consciously pursue certain missions or objectives and ignore others which might derail them. The formally adopted missions define the department's reasons for existing and determine the range of activities in which the department might engage, for example, patient counseling, third party negotiations, public relations activities, cash management, and data processing.

In addition, the department's mission will dictate to a large degree the kind of employee best suited to the department in terms of skills, experience, and education. Missions adopted by the patient account manager can also determine the complexity and formality of decision-making mechanisms as well as the type of internal systems and controls required.

Finally, the patient account department's mission determines how it relates to the hospital's external environment, including its patient population, community groups, other health care providers, government and regulatory agencies, and special interest groups that influence the successful accomplishment of the department's mission either directly or indirectly.

In establishing a departmental mission or revising an existing one, the patient account manager should realize the wide range of possible missions—all of which have definite implications for the long-range philosophical and operational character of the department. By confronting this issue at the outset, the patient account manager can anticipate difficulties and create operational mechanisms for resolving them.

Missions typically address the following issues:

- patient convenience and economics
- hospital convenience and economics
- hospital development
- service to the patient

Each of these issues has a spectrum of mission possibilities. A department may pursue several missions simultaneously or sequentially. In addition, a department may assign priorities for subsets of missions. Established missions should be routinely reviewed, modified, and updated to assure that the hospital is satisfying the needs of every segment of its market, for example, patients, physicians, employees, and community.

MISSIONS DEFINED

For illustration, the mission Memorial Hospital, Anytown, U.S.A., has developed for its patient business services department can be examined:

To render patient business (nonmedical) services to Memorial Hospital's patients and their third party guarantors, which will not only expedite the collection of cash for services rendered but also create an attitudinal environment that constantly enhances the hospital's image in the community and generates a sense of pride to the medical staff, nonmedical staff, and employees associated with the hospital; to assure the community that the hospital will produce sufficient cash resources to guarantee the hospital's financial viability and its readiness to meet the community's health care needs.

The following six objectives have been identified as essential in carrying out the department's mission:

1. to elevate and improve the status, quality, and quantity of business services to the hospital's patients
2. to be cost effective, without sacrificing quality of service
3. to assist and counsel patients in managing and meeting their financial obligations to the hospital
4. to minimize the hospital's losses due to bad debts and uncollectible accounts
5. to work with the other hospital departments and the medical staff in order to create an effective two-way communication system which will enhance and expedite reimbursement to the hospital and the physician
6. to accomplish these objectives in an environment that is efficient and pleasant for patients, medical staff, and hospital employees

The process of testing whether the department achieves these objectives and fulfills its mission is called performance evaluation. To make performance evaluation possible, the patient account manager should develop a formal management plan that includes the following:

- hospital policies
- operating procedures
- information systems
- required resources
- performance standards
- financial planning (budget)

Each of these components must be directed toward and complementary to the department's overall mission. The first four components will be discussed later in this chapter; performance standards will be covered in Chapter 5; and financial planning will be discussed in Chapter 6.

MANAGEMENT PLANNING DEFINED

Before discussing the methodology of effective management planning, an examination of Webster's definitions of management and planning may be useful. Webster's defines manage as "to handle, to control; to make and keep submissive; to alter by manipulation, to succeed in accomplishing; to continue; to direct or carry on business affairs; to achieve one's purpose."[4] The key words in this definition are:

- control
- manipulate
- succeed
- continue
- direct
- achieve

Webster's defines planning as "to plant, fix in place; a method of carrying out a design; a method of doing something; a detailed program of action; goal, aim; an orderly arrangement of parts of an overall design or objective."[5] The key words in this definition are:

- fix
- method
- design
- detailed program
- goal
- orderly arrangement

In conclusion, management planning is the process used by management to organize and to plan strategy in order to successfully achieve an identified mission and its set of objectives in an orderly and systematic way.

ORGANIZATIONAL DESIGN

Management planning begins with organizational design. A well-designed organization is necessary to implement the management plan. The management plan and organizational design should fit an individual manager's style.

In order to manage effectively, the patient account manager must first organize him- or herself and his or her subordinates. Seven steps comprise the organizational design planning process (see Figure 1–1):

Step 1. *Self-evaluation.* During this step, which might take a week or two, the manager relates his or her abilities and skills to the strategies, policies, and systems necessary to accomplish the department's mission.

Step 2. *Initial Documentation.* With his or her strengths and weaknesses in mind, the manager jots down ideas related to strategy, organizational design, resources, and systems. (Ideas should be written down every day as they occur.)

Step 3. *Organization.* The ideas collected up to this point should be organized in terms of the tasks required to achieve the department mission. This list should be in sequential order.

Step 4. *Preview.* After the initial plan has been developed, the manager should review it with his or her supervisors and subordinates who will be actively involved in its implementation, execution, or evaluation.

Step 5. *Formalization.* In this step, the manager incorporates all appropriate suggestions from Step 4 into a formal document that must be approved in writing by the hospital's chief executive officer or another appropriate supervising officer.

Step 6. *Implementation and Execution.* During this step, the manager and his or her supervisors implement the plan and manage the operations.

Step 7. *Review and Evaluation.* In this step, the manager and other appropriate individuals evaluate operating results in terms of pre-established performance standards. Review and evaluation should take place at least once a month, depending on the importance of the function being evaluated.

To assure maximum creativity and results, the manager should isolate him- or herself during Steps 2 and 3. The results of these "quiet times" will have a substantial impact on the method and organization of the department's operations. In completing Steps 2 and 3, the manager should try to be as open-minded, daring, and creative as possible, yet realistic. It is also wise not to expect to develop the ideal plan on the first attempt. Generally, many rewrites, additions, deletions, and revisions are necessary

8   PATIENT ACCOUNT MANAGEMENT

Figure 1-1 Seven Steps to a Successful Management Planning Process

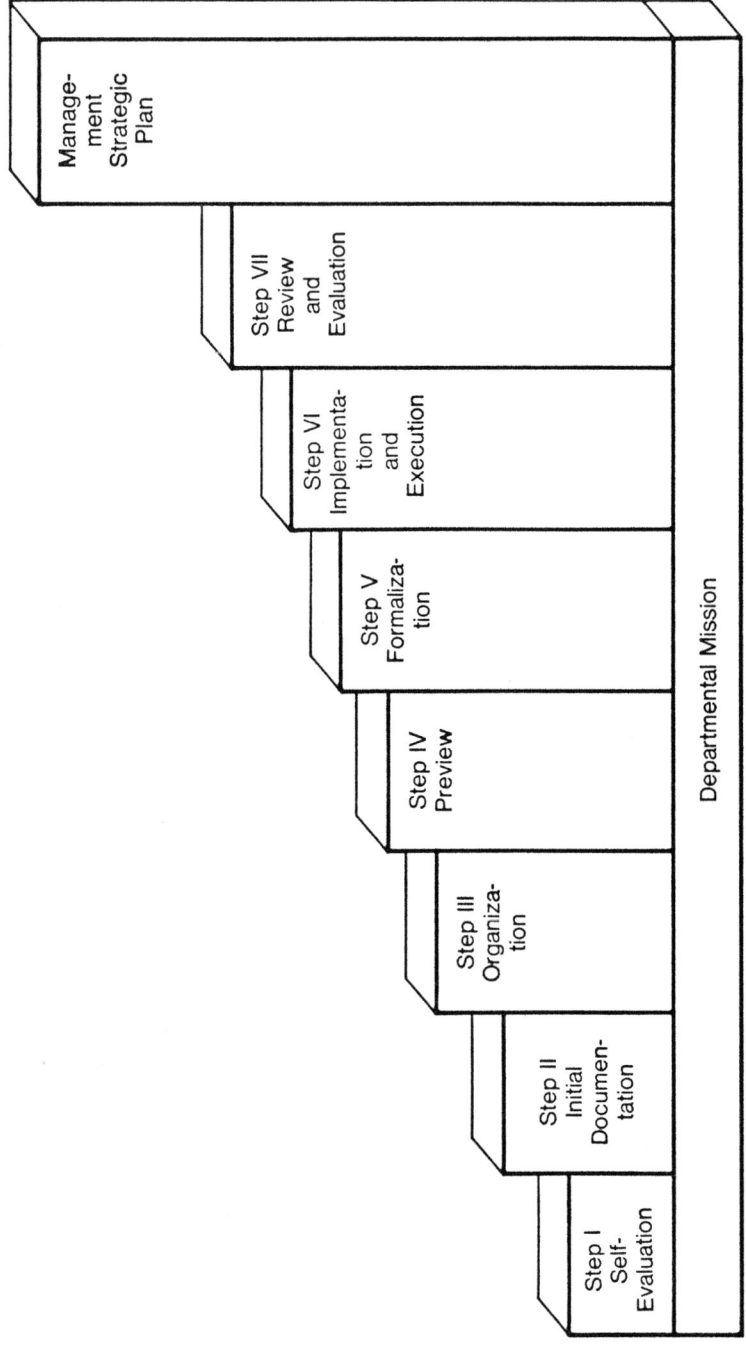

to produce a preliminary organizational plan ready for previewing (Step 4).

The patient account manager must adhere to three fundamental rules of organizational design in preparing the plan for the department. The first rule is to identify primary responsibility centers (for example, admitting, billing, collections, counseling, etc.) and to assign responsibility for each center to one individual. The individual's responsibility and standards of performance (production) must be well-defined (in writing) and mutually understood and accepted. In addition, the manager must delegate enough authority to the individual to provide sufficient latitude for effectively administering the area of responsibility.

The second rule is unity of command, which stipulates that an employee be responsible to only one supervisor. An employee should not be placed in the awkward position of having to decide which supervisor to report to. Frequently, an employee required to report to more than one supervisor becomes loyal to one supervisor at the expense of the other. At best, the employee will be ineffectively loyal to both supervisors.

The third rule deals with span of control, or the maximum number of subordinates any one supervisor can effectively supervise. A supervisor with too many subordinates runs the risk of either creating a bottleneck of indecision or making inappropriate decisions. The optimum number of subordinates reporting to one supervisor depends on several factors:

- the supervisor's ability to manage effectively;
- the financial or personnel impact of the supervisor's decisions on the department or the hospital;
- the number or frequency of decisions the supervisor must make; and
- the ability of the subordinates to manage themselves and allocate their time effectively.

Five to eight subordinates are generally considered to be a manageable number for a department manager or section supervisor to supervise directly.[6] Individuals who perform routine and repetitious tasks generally require less direct supervision; consequently, a supervisor should be able to manage as many as 25 such employees.

Figure 1–2 illustrates the traditional design of a patient business services department, and Figure 1–3 is an example of an organizational design which incorporates the patient service representative (PSR) system. Both charts depict organizational design:

10 PATIENT ACCOUNT MANAGEMENT

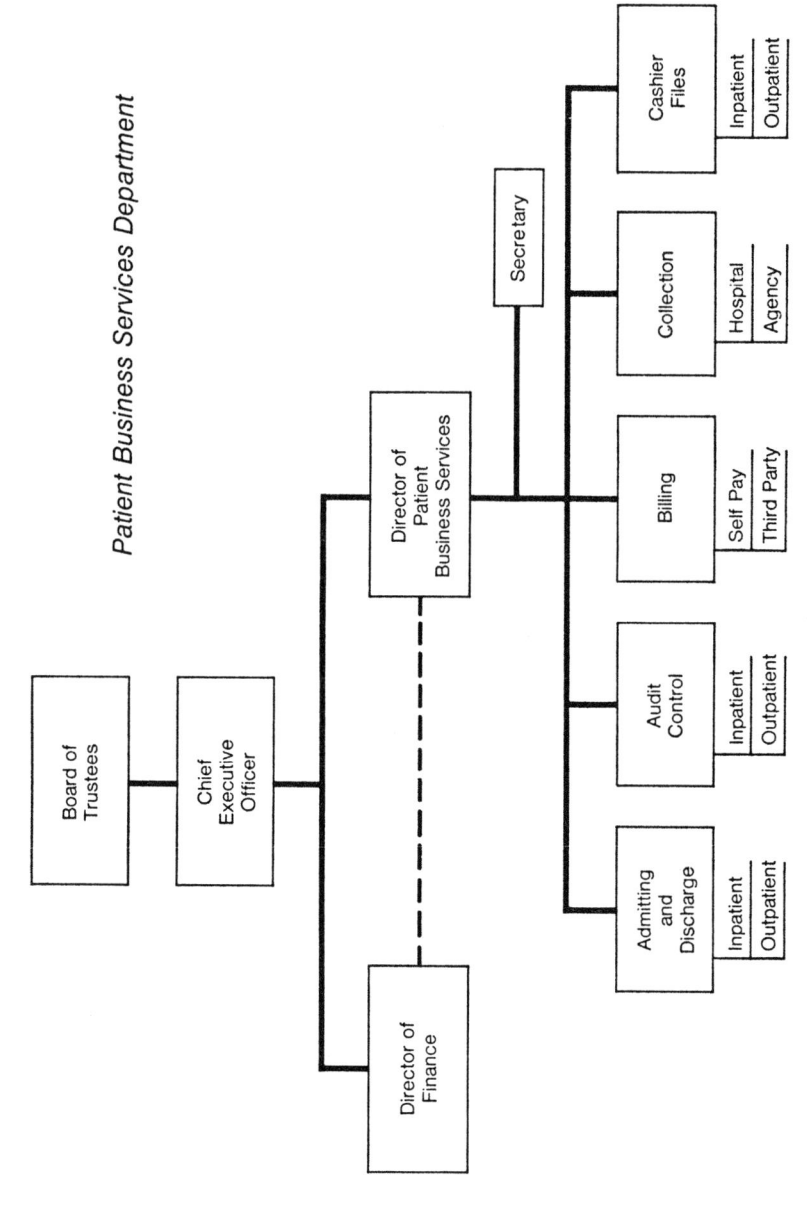

Figure 1-2 Traditional Organizational Design, Memorial Hospital, Anytown, U.S.A.

Patient Business Services Department 11

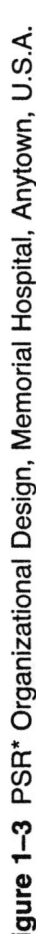

Figure 1-3 PSR* Organizational Design, Memorial Hospital, Anytown, U.S.A.

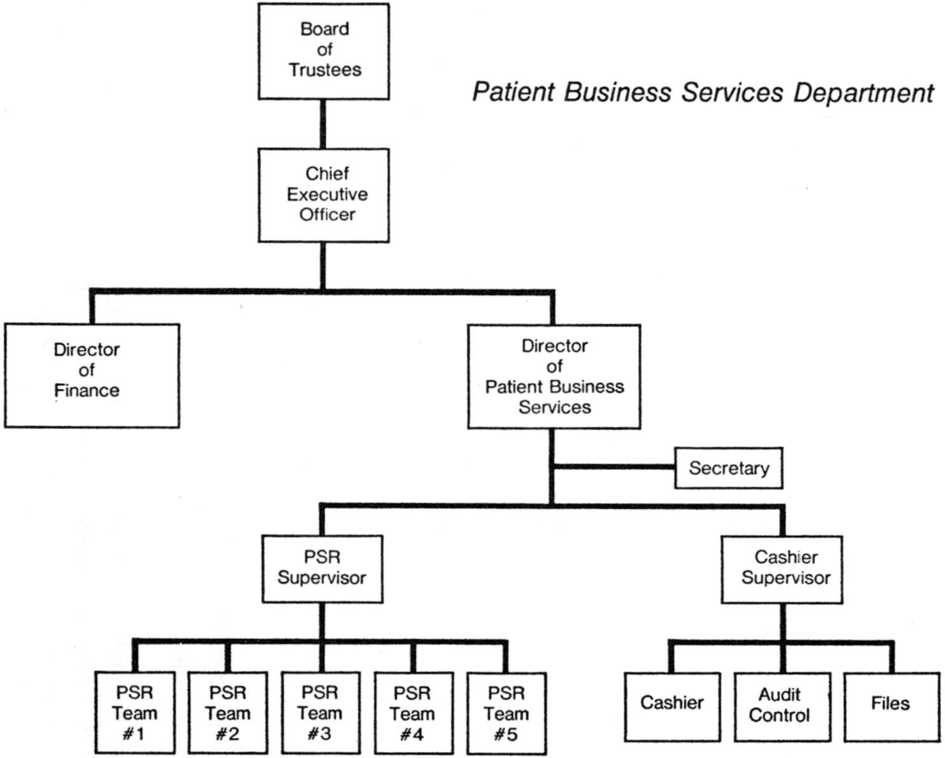

Patient Business Services Department

* Patient Service Representative

- delegation of responsibility
- unity of command
- span of control

Once the patient account manager has developed an organizational design for the department—keeping in mind that nothing is permanent at this point—the planning process continues. There are seven basic steps in the preliminary operational management planning process:

1. Identify specific goals and objectives that will achieve the department's mission.
2. Design the strategy to be used to attain specific goals and objectives.
3. Identify labor, nonlabor services and supplies, capital equipment, and financial resources required to implement the strategy.
4. Design an implementation plan that includes training and other start-up functions.
5. Develop an operational plan that includes policies, procedures, and methods.
6. Develop performance standards which can be used to monitor and evaluate operating results.
7. Develop a methodology and assign responsibility for feedback and evaluating actual operations in terms of performance standards and taking necessary corrective measures.

Defining the department's specific objectives is one of the most important steps in the management planning process. There are two basic approaches to setting departmental objectives:

1. unilateral
2. multilateral

In the unilateral ("Theory X") approach, planning and, specifically, objective setting, is done entirely by the manager with little, if any, input from subordinates. The multilateral ("Theory Y" and/or "Z") approach, on the other hand, calls for planning and establishment of objectives to be done by the people who have the ultimate responsibility for making the plan work. If planning time is limited, and some stopgap decisions must be made, the unilateral approach will frequently effect desirable short-term results. However, the involvement approach that is part of multilateral planning generally improves employee morale and productivity over the long term.

Once objectives have been identified and priorities have been established, the strategy required to accomplish these objectives must be determined. Again, a multilateral approach generally produces the best long-term results because of its synergistic effect. Usually, it requires more time than the unilateral method, but the results tend to be worth the extra time required.

Identification of resources is the next step. These resources include the following:

- labor
- nonlabor supplies and services
- capital equipment and facilities
- money

This step requires the patient account manager to assess the resources the hospital already possesses, as well as any additional resources needed to implement the strategic plan. A corresponding financial requirement plan (budget) is a critical management tool in this process. The budget is discussed in Chapter 6. Along with the financial plan, a cost-benefit analysis of each program should be completed so that management can evaluate the economic and social feasibility of the program. Every program should stand on its own merits.

The implementation and execution of the plan is substantially easier if thoughtful consideration has been given to the first five steps in the management planning process. A well thought-out, formal plan makes the decision-making process almost automatic.

Actually, the review and evaluation process starts before the plan is even implemented. Performance standards are established as part of the first five steps in the management planning process. The terms "performance standards" and "production standards" are often used interchangeably. This author prefers the term "performance standard." According to Webster's, performance is "the execution of an action; something accomplished, the fulfillment of a claim, promise or request."[7]

Webster's defines production as "total output, especially of a commodity or industry."[8] Thus, a performance standard is a reasonable quantitative measurement or level of work that management expects to be accomplished over a specific period of time. Again, a multilateral approach to establishment of performance standards usually proves most effective. Management expectations must be realistic and attainable. Also, they must be reassessed periodically to ensure that they are producing the desired results. Chapter 5 describes the development and use of performance standards in considerable detail.

As the review and evaluation process is being designed, it is important to make sure that it incorporates procedures that management can use to systematically and continually compare results to standards and take appropriate corrective measures.

DELEGATION OF AUTHORITY

An adjunct function of the management planning process is the delegation of authority. There are some responsibilities the patient account manager cannot delegate including leadership, coordination, and evaluation. Staff assistants may help the manager carry out these duties, but the manager is ultimately responsible. Thus, delegation means the assignment of only part of the manager's work. Some managers are reluctant to delegate work because they believe they will lose control; other managers delegate work and forget about it. Both approaches are dangerous. In the first case, the manager is not developing a management team. In the second, the manager has abdicated a responsibility with no feedback or accountability.

According to W. H. Nesbitt of Westinghouse Electric Corporation, there are six degrees of delegation:

1. Take action—no further contact with me is needed.
2. Take action—let me know what you did.
3. Look into the problem—let me know what you intend to do, and do it unless I say not to.
4. Look into the problem—let me know what you intend to do, and delay action until I give approval.
5. Look into the problem—let me know the alternative actions, including the pros and cons of each, and recommend one for my approval.
6. Look into the problem—give me all the facts, and I will decide what to do.[9]

At each level, the manager is delegating some degree of fact finding, decision making, and action.

Sherman offers these four general guidelines for successful delegation:

1. As far as possible, delegate a job by the results you want and not by the methods to be used. Your subordinate should be free to do the job his or her own way—as long as his or her actions do not violate overall policy or cause other major problems. This approach works most effectively when performance standards have been set.

2. Give the employee all the relevant information he or she needs to perform the delegated work. Establish a climate of free and open discussion, but make it clear that you expect completed staff work.
3. Delegate work only to qualified people. You must understand the abilities and limitations of your subordinates to do this effectively. Remember, the question is not primarily whether the subordinate can do the job as well as you, but whether he or she can do it adequately, whether doing it is desirable from the standpoint of the subordinate's development, or whether you should be spending your time on more important matters.
4. Establish controls (feedback mechanisms) that will alert you to difficulties early.[10]

Ray Boedecker of International Business Machines (IBM) has identified ten common mistakes a manager can make in delegating:

1. Failing to delegate enough.
2. Delegating by formula.
3. Failing to keep communication lines open.
4. Failing to make the assignment stick.
5. Failing to define the assignments.
6. Failing to delegate enough authority to do the job.
7. Being too narrow in delegation.
8. Failing to keep up-to-date on delegated jobs.
9. Failing to allow for mistakes.
10. Failing to close the loop on delegation.[11]

In summary, assembling, organizing, and developing an effective management team is undoubtedly one of the most important functions of the patient account manager. When Andrew Carnegie was asked what he attributed his success to, he responded, "I hire the right people." In fact, the responsibility of developing an effective management team can be carried one step further; the patient account manager has the additional responsibility of assisting his or her subordinates in expanding and developing their skills, capabilities, and horizons.

JOB ANALYSIS

An integral part of the management planning process is job analysis. This function requires the patient account manager to thoroughly analyze the types of tasks delegated to each job or position in the organizational design, and the personal qualities, experience, and education needed to perform these tasks.

For example, if one were to analyze the patient service representative (PSR) position, the following functions might be identified:

- Conduct preadmission and/or admission processing with inpatients being admitted to the hospital or outpatients receiving services from the hospital.
- Attempt to collect cash from patients according to hospital policies.
- Initiate billing to either the patient and/or the third party guarantor.
- Conduct follow-up billing on unpaid accounts.
- Prepare uncollectible accounts for referral to outside collection agencies and maintain a control file for these accounts.
- Serve as the patient's own hospital representative and advisor on all issues concerning the patient's account receivable while he or she is in the hospital and until the account is totally settled.
- Obtain a firm commitment from the patient or responsible party before or at discharge concerning the method and time payment schedule for paying the account in full.
- Work with the patient, medical staff, and other hospital personnel to assure prompt and full payment of the account receivable.
- Serve as the hospital's goodwill ambassador and counselor to the patient and the community in order to enhance the hospital's image.

Some of the qualifications for this position might include:

- Education: High school graduate.
- Experience: Six months to one year.
- Technical skills: Ability to type at least 40 words per minute and use calculator and telephone.
- Personality traits: Ability to meet and communicate with people easily; self-starter who can adjust quickly from one task to another; ability to keep information confidential.

JOB DESCRIPTION

Job analysis is the first step in writing a job description and developing performance standards (see Chapter 5). The typical job description contains 14 key pieces of information:

1. name of hospital
2. job title
3. department
4. immediate supervisor
5. job code number
6. chart of accounts number
7. job or labor grade
8. primary job function
9. specific job function
10. job qualifications
11. performance standards
12. date job description was written or revised
13. name and title of officer approving job description
14. date of approval

Figure 1-4 is an example of a job description format. This format is unique because it requires that each identified task has a performance standard. In this case, a performance standard means that a certain number of activities must be properly completed within a pre-established time period.

A job description serves the following three purposes:

1. It assists the manager or supervisor in identifying the basis or common ground upon which an employee's performance can be evaluated.
2. It serves as a basis for evaluating the qualifications of a prospective employee.
3. It assists the employee in evaluating his or her performance.

Job descriptions must be reviewed and approved by the appropriate supervisor. They should not be considered permanent but should be reviewed constantly to assure management that work has been appropriately delegated according to the needs of the hospital and the systems and procedures that have been established. It is especially important to continually review and evaluate performance standards.

SUMMARY

The management planning process applied to the organization of the patient business services department of a hospital requires a considerable amount of the patient account manager's time, forethought, and examination. As with any application of the management planning process, the patient account manager must:

18   PATIENT ACCOUNT MANAGEMENT

Figure 1–4 Sample Job Description Form, Memorial Hospital, Anytown, U.S.A.

JOB DESCRIPTION

JOB TITLE _____ JOB NUMBER _____

DEPARTMENT _____ JOB LABOR GRADE _____

IMMEDIATE SUPERVISOR _____ CHART OF ACCOUNT NO. _____

PRIMARY FUNCTION:

SPECIFIC FUNCTIONS	PERFORMANCE STANDARDS

JOB QUALIFICATIONS:

  EDUCATION:

  EXPERIENCE:

  TECHNICAL SKILLS:

  PERSONALITY TRAITS:

  CONFIDENTIALITY:

DATE APPROVED: _____ 19 _____

APPROVED BY _____ TITLE _____

- identify the mission and related goals and objectives
- plan strategy to meet these goals and objectives
- identify resources required to accomplish these goals and objectives
- establish performance standards before operations begin
- assign responsibility to monitor and evaluate actual performance in terms of established performance standards
- establish a feedback system and assign responsibility for taking corrective measures

There is no single most effective method to use. The approach that fits one manager's style could be disastrous for another. To be effective, the patient account manager should use the management planning approach that is the most comfortable and practicable.

NOTES

1. Harold Koontz and Cyril O'Donnell, *Essentials of Management* (New York, NY: McGraw-Hill Book Company, 1974), p. 1.
2. Douglas McGregor, *The Human Side of Enterprise* (New York, NY: McGraw-Hill Book Company, 1960), pp. 33–48.
3. William G. Ouchi, *Theory Z: How American Business Can Meet the Japanese Challenge* (Reading, Mass.: Addison-Wesley Publishing Co., 1981), p. 43.
4. *Webster's Seventh New Collegiate Dictionary* (Springfield, Mass.: G. & C. Merriam Co., 1961), p. 513.
5. Ibid., p. 396.
6. Allen G. Herkimer, Jr., *Understanding Hospital Financial Management* (Germantown, Md.: Aspen Systems Corp., 1978), p. 27.
7. *Webster's Seventh New Collegiate Dictionary*, p. 627.
8. Ibid., p. 679.
9. Harvey Sherman, *How Much Should You Delegate?* (New York: American Management Association, 1966), pp. 4–5.
10. Ibid., pp. 5–6.
11. Ray F. Boedecker, *Why Delegation Goes Wrong* (New York: American Management Association, 1964), pp. 1–5.

Chapter 2
The Use of Standard Plans

The patient account manager cannot manage effectively without clearly written, definitive standard plans governing each departmental function. The distinctive characteristic of a standard plan is that the same decision and action may be used and reused; it establishes a continuing pattern for dealing with everyday normal situations, thus enabling the manager and his or her staff to devote more time to unusual or difficult situations and to any procedural changes they wish to implement.

Standard plans can be divided into three major categories:

- policies
- procedures
- methods

These categories will be examined to determine their use and benefits for the patient account department. Organizational structure, too, may be considered a standard plan inasmuch as the assignment of tasks and the relationships established provide a continuing frame of reference to guide the patient account managers and their staffs in their daily activities.

POLICIES

A policy may be defined as a general plan of action that guides hospital personnel in their conduct and daily operations. Policies are set by the governing board and are implemented by the administrator, the director of finance, and the manager of patient accounts. Policies should be reviewed periodically to be certain that they are current and that the position or function to which a policy applies has not been changed or eliminated.

Within the guidelines of each policy, a procedure for the function it governs should be developed. It is important to recognize the difference between a policy and a procedure; a policy must be explicit in stating the hospital's position regarding the function to which it refers. A collection policy, for example, may be formulated based upon the following questions:

- Will the hospital use a preadmission system?
- Will the hospital require prepayment at admission?
- When is the patient's ability to pay established?
- When is the primary collection effort made?
- When does the hospital expect payment in full?
- Will the hospital charge interest on unpaid balances?
- When is an account considered delinquent?
- When is an account considered uncollectible?
- When is an account referred to an outside collection agency?
- Will the hospital permit the use of liens, attorneys, small claims court, etc.?
- Will the hospital give cash discounts?
- When is an account categorized as a bad debt?

The answer to these questions should determine the hospital's collection policies; these should be approved by the governing board, circulated to appropriate persons, and implemented by the manager of patient accounts and his or her department.

PROCEDURES

The distinction between policies, procedures, and methods is not always clear cut: a policy typically covers a basic issue or a broad area; a procedure or method normally deals with the way the function or task is carried out. This distinction between the broader aspects of an operating situation and the more detailed and specific considerations is useful in planning because it emphasizes a different viewpoint.[1]

Effective managers give appropriate and equal consideration to both policies and procedures; distinguishing between policies and procedures is necessary to the delegation process. In common usage procedures and methods are frequently used interchangeably. However, for this review, procedures will imply a series of steps, often taken by different individuals;

whereas, methods are concerned with only a single operation or workplace.[2]

A standard procedure should ensure that appropriate, complete information flows to the appropriate individuals needing the data and that each person involved in the process understands what he or she is responsible for. One dictionary defines procedure as "a series of steps followed in a regular order." When this regular order of steps becomes established as routine, the task of management is significantly simplified.

Written procedures are usually in one of two forms:

- step-by-step narration
- flow chart

A step-by-step narration of a hospital preadmitting procedure may be as follows:

Step 1. Physician's office notifies admitting office of pending admission.
Step 2. Preadmitting clerk obtains name, address, and telephone number of patient; also obtains admitting diagnosis.
Step 3. Preadmitting clerk contacts patient by telephone; obtains complete and accurate demographic and financial information.
Step 4. Preadmitting clerk (or insurance verifier) contacts payment guarantor to verify amount of insurance coverage.
Step 5. After verifying coverage, clerk telephones patient again. If insurance coverage is inadequate, clerk informs patient of hospital's requirements for advance payment, or payment in full by discharge.
Step 6. Preadmitting clerk informs patient of time he or she is expected in admitting office.

The preadmitting policy governing this procedure was determined, in part, from answers to questions referring to a collection policy and to questions that were asked and answered before an admitting policy was written. This step-by-step narrative procedure can be illustrated on a flow chart as illustrated in Figure 2–1.

Many procedures require transferring information to various persons or departments in written form. Whenever this is necessary, design of the standard forms that will be used becomes an important part of the procedure. Confusion can be reduced if forms are designed to be uniform in size with clearly defined lines and spaces for recording essential information. Properly designed forms facilitate accuracy, permit rapid use and verification, and standardize the record storage requirements. Color coding

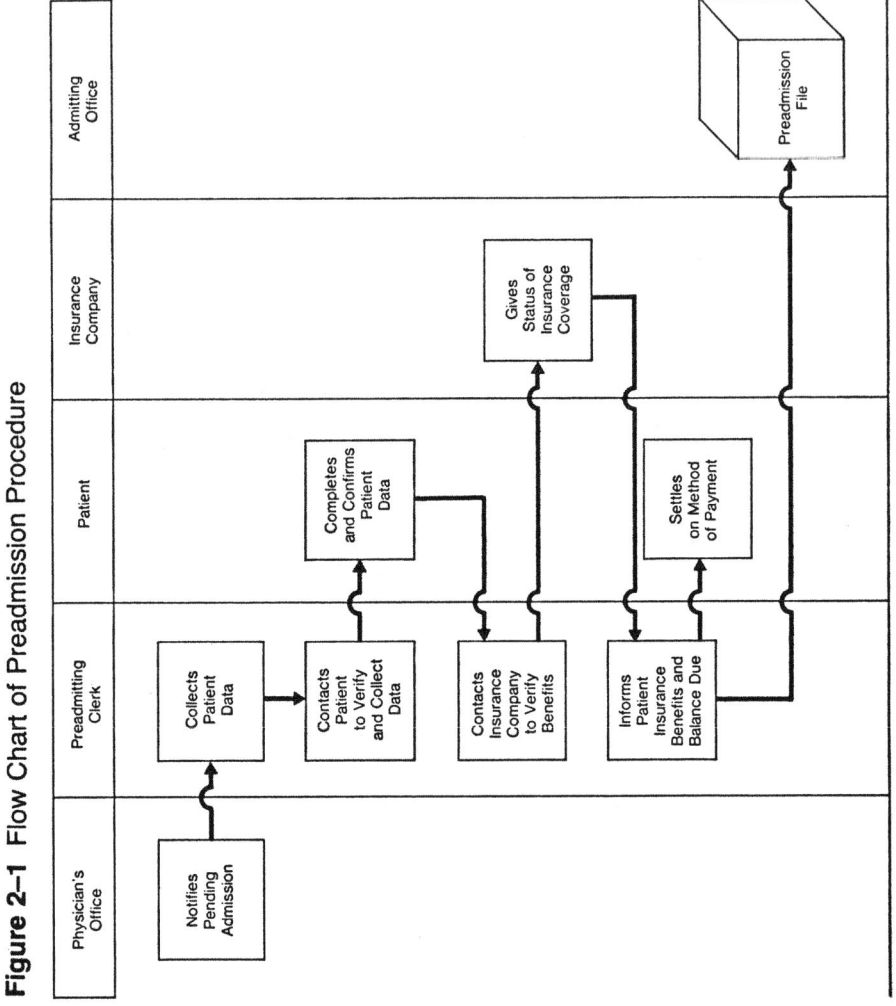

Figure 2-1 Flow Chart of Preadmission Procedure

a multipart form helps to assure that all designated users will receive the correct copy.

METHODS

A method differs from a procedure in that it deals with one single operation only. Defining one specific method for use assumes that there is only one most efficient method for a particular job or situation; testing and experience are necessary before the best method is determined. Part of the patient account manager's responsibility is training personnel and maintaining standard operating conditions within the department; within these conditions, every employee is expected to perform according to an approved method.

Standard methods contribute to the efficiency of the department and to the maintenance of the desired level of quality of work. Standard methods may be detailed or general to allow for adjustment to existing conditions.

A method for use in the preadmitting procedure might be a prepared set of questions and responses; another might be a prepared "script" for talking with discharged patients who are delinquent in payments. Standard methods that have been tested for effectiveness and that result in these procedures can assure collection of the complete accurate data the function demands.

BENEFITS OF STANDARD PLANS

The three types of standard plans—policies, procedures, and methods—serve as a guide for the patient account manager and his or her staff to uniformly implement departmental functions and to maintain them consistently. The development and use of these standards provoke some practical questions:

- When should they be used?
- How specific and detailed should they be?

The answers to these questions become apparent when the patient account manager recognizes the benefits of using written standard operating policies, procedures, and methods:

- Standards result in less time being required for crisis management; decision making becomes virtually automatic.

- Standards make maintaining performance and work quality easier because, theoretically, the one most efficient method has been identified.
- Standards, together with a well-designed organizational structure, facilitate delegating authority and responsibility.
- Standards are the basis of the patient account manager's evaluation of performance by an individual, a group, a system, or subsystem in the department.
- Standards ensure that interdepartmental and intradepartmental activities will be conducted consistently and efficiently.

NOTES

1. David R. Hampton, Charles E. Summer, and Ross A. Weber, *Organizational Behavior and the Practice of Management* (Glenview, Ill.: Scott, Foresman & Company, 1968), p. 622.
2. Ibid., p. 623.

Chapter 3

The Hospital Accounting Process

The quality and integrity of the financial and statistical information the patient account manager uses is the responsibility of the hospital's chief financial officer and accounting staff. The patient account manager, however, is responsible for interpreting this information.

Seawell states that, unlike the natural laws which govern the physical sciences, the basic concepts and principles of accounting—which are sometimes called postulates, rules, conventions, or standards—are the result of a continuing evolutionary process. They are subject to periodic reevaluation and possible change. They can be modified or even discarded in response to changes in economic or social conditions, technology, methods of conducting economic activity, or user demands for more serviceable information. This absence of absolute permanency is not entirely undesirable according to Seawell. Describing accounting as an art, not a science, he points out that it must change as its environment and the needs of its users change.[1]

This chapter will acquaint the patient account manager with the basic concepts and principles of hospital accounting to improve his or her understanding of key financial reports and how they are generated.

Hospital accounting is based on three fundamental principles:

1. double entry bookkeeping
2. accrual accounting
3. fund accounting

It should be noted, however, that one of these principles, fund accounting, seems to be used less now than previously.

DOUBLE ENTRY BOOKKEEPING

The underlying theory of double entry bookkeeping is that every accounting transaction requires a minimum of two entries or changes in the accounting records—thus, the name, double entry. The basic principle of double entry bookkeeping is:

For every debit there must be an equal and offsetting credit.

Debits and credits are the terms used to distinguish one side of the double entry from the other. Debits are recorded on the left side of the ledger, while credits are recorded on the right side, as illustrated in the T-account format below:

Debit	Credit

The abbreviations for these terms are:

Debit: (DR)
Credit: (CR)

The basic principles for using debits and credits in key accounts are shown in Table 3-1. The important fact to remember is that there must be equal and offsetting debits and credits in every accounting transaction. This does not mean that only one debit and only one credit can be made at a time.

The two basic types of accounting entries or transactions are: (1) single, and (2) compound. The single entry records transactions in only two accounts. For example, one debit entry and one credit entry are made in the journal with the debit listed first and the credit indented:

	Debit	*Credit*
Cash	$1,000	
Accounts Receivable		$1,000

To record cash received on Accounts Receivable from the Cash Receipts Journal.

The Hospital Accounting Process 29

Table 3-1 Double Entry Bookkeeping Impact Matrix

Account Description	Debit Impact	Credit Impact
Asset	Increases Value	Decreases Value
Liability	Decreases Payable	Increases Payable
Capital or Equity	Decreases Worth	Increases Worth
Revenue	Decreases Income	Increases Income
Expense	Increases Costs	Decreases Costs

In T-accounts, these entries would appear as follows:

Cash		Accounts Receivable	
$1,000			$1,000

The compound entry records transactions in more than two accounts, but the total dollar debits equal the total dollar credits as illustrated below:

Accounts Receivable $1,000
   Nursing Revenue $600
   Surgery Revenue 150
   Laboratory Revenue 100
   Radiology Revenue.. 100
   Pharmacy Revenue 50

To record revenues generated from Accounts Receivable to the Revenue Journal.

These entries would be made in T-accounts as follows:

Accounts Receivable		Nursing Revenue	
$1,000			$600

Surgery Revenue	Laboratory Revenue
$150	$100

Radiology Revenue	Pharmacy Revenue
$100	$50

These examples illustrate the use of double entry bookkeeping in the hospital accounting process. It is important to note that in both the single and compound transactions, debits always equal credits.

ACCRUAL ACCOUNTING

The accrual concept of accounting requires that revenues, expenses, and other related transactions be recognized and recorded as they are incurred, regardless of the related cash flow. The accrual concept is exactly the opposite of the cash concept of accounting under which revenues and expenses are recognized and recorded only when the cash is actually received or disbursed.

In the past, hospitals used cash accounting, despite the fact that cash accounting does not accurately indicate a hospital's financial condition. In the cash accounting system, revenues are not recorded until cash is received from the patient; therefore, revenues for a given accounting period may be overstated or understated. Similarly, a hospital may not have enough cash to pay current obligations, so expenses represented by the unpaid vendor invoices are not recorded. As a result, operating expenses for the accounting period may be understated. Conversely, if all vendors are paid up to date, expenses could be overstated.

When the cash accounting system is used, the revenue and expense statement might report a break-even financial condition (see Table 3-2), when in fact the hospital is operating at a loss because it is indebted to vendors and a considerable amount of accounts receivable are uncollected. In this case, the revenue and expense statement would be more accurately described as a cash flow statement (see Table 3-3).

The two missing elements or accounts in the cash accounting system are: (1) accounts receivable, and (2) accounts payable. Incorporating these primary accounts into the accounting system in effect turns it into an accrual accounting system because revenues and expenses are recognized and recorded during the accounting period in which they are earned or incurred.

Table 3–2 Revenue and Expense Statement Using the Cash Accounting Method

Memorial Hospital, Anytown, U.S.A.
Revenue and Expense Statement
For the Three-Month Period Ending September 30, 19x1

This Month		Year-to-Date
$100,000	Revenue	$300,000
99,000	Less: Expense	299,000
$ 1,000	Profit (Loss)	$ 1,000

Table 3–3 Cash Flow Statement

Memorial Hospital, Anytown, U.S.A.
Cash Flow Statement
For the Three-Month Period Ending September 30, 19x1

This Month		Year-to-Date
$100,000	Cash Received	$300,000
99,000	Less: Cash Disbursed	299,000
$ 1,000	Cash on Hand	$ 1,000

To illustrate the month's transactions in Tables 3–2 and 3–3 using the accrual accounting system, the following account entries are made:

Cash $100,000
Accounts Receivable.. $100,000

To record cash received on Patient Accounts Receivable during the month from the Cash Receipts Journal.

Accounts Payable................................ $99,000
Cash $99,000

To record cash disbursed on Accounts Payable during the month from the Cash Disbursements Journal.

Accounts Receivable.......................... $150,000
    Revenue $150,000

To record revenue charged during the month from the Revenue Journal.

Expenses $125,000
    Accounts Payable $125,000

To record expenses incurred during the month from the Purchase Journal.

The T-account entries would be made as follows:

Cash		Accounts Receivable	
(1) $100,000	(2) $99,000	(3) $150,000	(1) $100,000
Balance $1,000		Balance $50,000	

Accounts Payable		Revenue	
(2) $99,000	(4) $125,000		(3) $150,000
	Balance $26,000		

Expenses	
(4) $125,000	

To illustrate further the impact of the difference in the two accounting systems, Table 3–4 provides a comparative analysis of the month's activity.

The matching of revenue and expense is an integral function of the accrual accounting system. Not only must revenues and expenses associated with a specific accounting period be reported together, but deductions from gross revenue, such as bad debts, contractual allowances, policy discounts, and other adjustments to generated revenues, must also be reported together to assure a true matching of revenues and expenses.

Table 3-4 Comparative Analysis of Cash and Accrual Methods

Memorial Hospital, Anytown, U.S.A.
Statement of Operation
For the Month Ending September 30, 19xx

	Cash Method	Accrual Method
Revenue	$100,000	$150,000
Expense	99,000	125,000
Profit (Loss)	$ 1,000	$ 25,000
Supplemental Information:		
Cash	$ 1,000	$ 1,000
Accounts Receivable	Not Recorded	50,000
Accounts Payable	Not Recorded	(26,000)
Total	$ 1,000	$ 25,000

FUND ACCOUNTING

Fund accounting distinguishes traditional hospital accounting from the accounting systems used in most other businesses. When the American Hospital Association (AHA) originally recommended fund accounting in its publication *Chart of Accounts for Hospitals*, many hospitals were receiving substantial amounts of money in the form of donations, grants, and other restricted monies. It was imperative that hospitals record and manage these funds in compliance with their individual legal restrictions. Hence, most hospitals came to use fund accounting.

The principle of fund accounting requires that each fund be segregated into independent, self-balancing groups of accounts. In addition, each fund must have its own balance sheet accounts, that is, assets, liabilities, and fund balance. Hospital funds are divided into two major groups: (1) unrestricted, and (2) restricted. Unrestricted funds have no external restrictions on their use and purpose; they can be used for any purpose chosen by the hospital board and/or administration. Restricted funds are funds whose use is restricted by the donors to specific purposes. In some cases, such as endowment funds, the original donation is restricted, but income from investing it can be used for operations or other purposes.

The Annual Hospital Report (AHR) and the Medicare reporting system proposed by the Health Care Financing Administration (HCFA) suggest that funds be categorized as:[2]

- unrestricted funds—operating
- restricted funds—specific purpose fund
- restricted funds—endowment fund
- restricted funds—plant replacement and expansion fund

Accounting procedures for funds can become complex because of the "due to" and "due from" accounts necessary to assure that each fund is always in balance. Another problem encountered in fund accounting is the fact that the resulting financial statements may be misleading to the user. The user who does not look at all of a hospital's balance sheets is aware of only part of the hospital's total assets and liabilities. Therefore, it is imperative that the hospital's financial condition be reported in a consolidated balance sheet similar to the one shown in Exhibit 3–1.

PREREQUISITES OF AN ACCOUNTING SYSTEM

Certain key management tools are prerequisites for successful operation of an accounting system:

- organizational chart
- chart of accounts

Exhibit 3–1 Consolidated Balance Sheet

Memorial Hospital, Anytown, U.S.A.
Consolidated Balance Sheet
As of September 30, 19x1

	Total	Operating Fund	Specific Purpose Fund	Endowment Fund	Plant Fund
Assets					
Current Assets	$ xxx	$ xxx	$ xxx	$ xxx	$ xxx
Fixed Assets	xxx	xxx	xxx	xxx	xxx
Total Assets	$ xxx	$ xxx	$ xxx	$ xxx	$ xxx
Liabilities and Capital					
Current Liabilities	$ xxx	$ xxx	$ xxx	$ xxx	$ xxx
Fixed Liabilities	xxx	xxx	xxx	xxx	xxx
Total Liabilities	$ xxx	$ xxx	$ xxx	$ xxx	$ xxx
Capital	xxx	xxx	xxx	xxx	xxx
Total Liabilities and Capital	$ xxx	$ xxx	$ xxx	$ xxx	$ xxx

- documented proof
- journals and ledgers

Organizational Chart

An effective organization may be defined as a group of individuals who cooperate successfully to achieve a common objective.[3] In building an effective management team, one must consider:

- the organizational structure, that is, the grouping of functions that most effectively promotes cooperation and determination of the optimal relationship among those groups
- the proper delegation of responsibility and authority to all managers and supervisors
- the selection of the right people for every job

The final test of the effectiveness of an organization is its ability to:

- provide the services required of it
- provide those services at minimal cost without sacrificing quality
- develop competent personnel

The organizational chart puts all these factors together in a formal, easily understood format that identifies:

- functions
- lines of authority and communication
- delegation of responsibility

In addition, the organizational chart serves as the basis for identifying and assigning departmental account numbers from the hospital's chart of accounts.

Chart of Accounts

The AHA's *Chart of Accounts for Hospitals* defines the chart of accounts as a list of account titles with numerical symbols designed for the compiling of financial data concerning the assets, liabilities, equity, revenues, and expenses of an enterprise. According to AHA, the classifications in a hospital's chart of accounts should correspond to the divisions of responsibility shown in its current organizational chart. Because no two hospitals are, or necessarily should be, organized in exactly the same way, no two hospitals will have identical charts of accounts.[4]

HCFA does not agree with the AHA position. Under the authority of the Medicare-Medicaid Antifraud and Abuse Amendments (PL 95-142, Section 19), HCFA developed the AHR, which requires hospitals to ". . . employ such chart of accounts definitions, principles and statistics as the Secretary [Department of Health and Human Services] may prescribe in order to reach a uniform reconciliation of financial and statistical data for specified uniform reports to be provided to the Secretary."[5] All hospitals receiving reimbursement under the Medicare and Medicaid programs (except for Christian Science Sanitoria) must conform to this reporting system.

Aware that hospitals have reporting and accounting needs other than meeting the requirements of federal and state programs, HCFA has designed the AHR so that it includes a reclassification system that will permit hospitals to reclassify information generated by internal systems for AHR reporting.[6]

Since the AHR is intended to capture cost and utilization data on a functional cost center basis, it conflicts directly with the concept of responsibility accounting and budgetary control. A responsibility accounting and budgetary control system accumulates and communicates to the responsible managers forecasted and actual financial and statistical data relating to revenues and controllable expenses classified according to the hospital's organizational chart departments that generate the revenue and are responsible for causing the expenses. The functional accounting system mandated by AHR requires that revenues and expenses be grouped by functions, such as patient accounting, housekeeping, and laboratory, regardless of who is personally responsible for these revenues and expenses in terms of the organizational chart.

Figure 3–1 shows how an organizational chart and a chart of accounts may be linked by expanding the traditional organizational design shown in Figure 1–1 and using the AHA chart of accounts numerical coding system for fiscal and administrative services.[7]

Documented Proof

Before an accounting transaction can be recorded, the accountant must have documented proof that supports the entry into the accounting system. Documented proof is necessary in order to protect the integrity of the entry and to provide evidence for internal and external audits.

There has been much controversy, especially in the area of capital assets, over what financial value should be entered in the hospital's books of

The Hospital Accounting Process 37

Figure 3–1 Organizational Chart

Memorial Hospital, Anytown, U.S.A.
Organizational Chart
Fiscal and Administrative Services

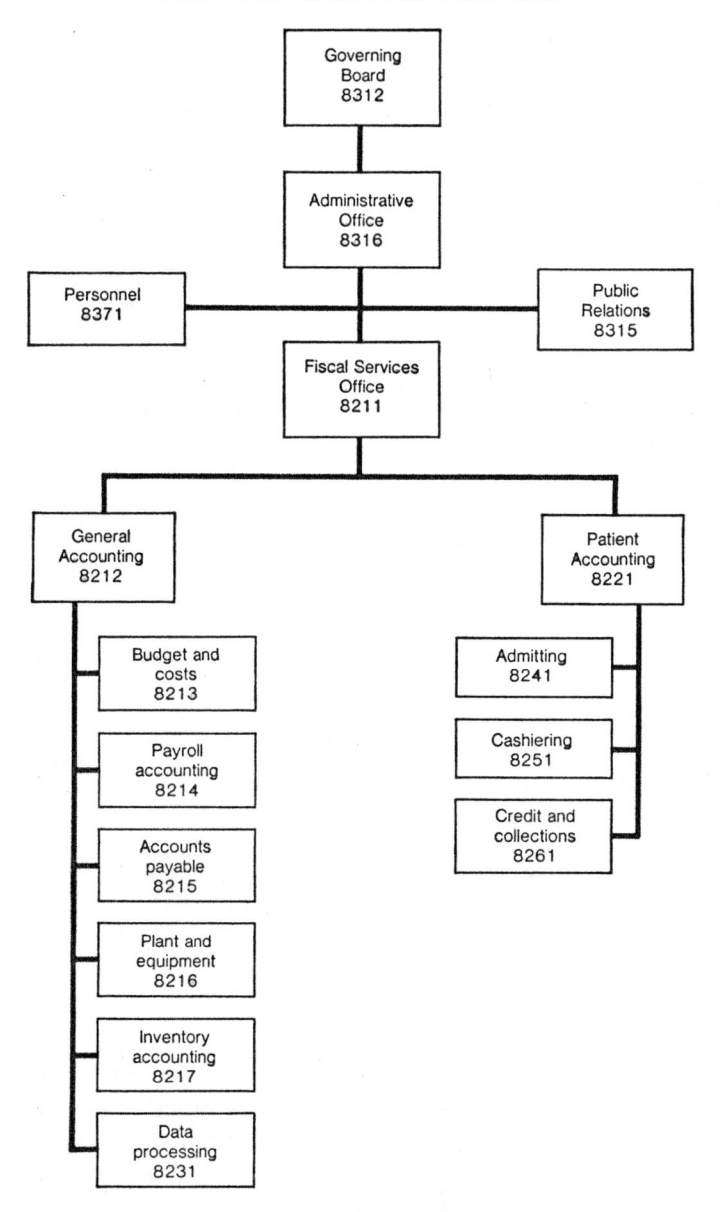

```
                    ┌─────────────┐
                    │  Governing  │
                    │    Board    │
                    │    8312     │
                    └──────┬──────┘
                           │
                    ┌──────┴──────┐
                    │Administrative│
                    │   Office    │
                    │    8316     │
                    └──────┬──────┘
        ┌──────────────────┼──────────────────┐
  ┌─────┴─────┐            │            ┌─────┴─────┐
  │ Personnel │            │            │  Public   │
  │   8371    │            │            │ Relations │
  │           │            │            │   8315    │
  └───────────┘            │            └───────────┘
                    ┌──────┴──────┐
                    │Fiscal Services│
                    │   Office    │
                    │    8211     │
                    └──────┬──────┘
              ┌────────────┴────────────┐
      ┌───────┴───────┐         ┌───────┴───────┐
      │    General    │         │    Patient    │
      │  Accounting   │         │  Accounting   │
      │     8212      │         │     8221      │
      └───────┬───────┘         └───────┬───────┘
              │                         │
         ┌────┴────────┐           ┌────┴────────┐
         │ Budget and  │           │  Admitting  │
         │    costs    │           │    8241     │
         │    8213     │           └─────────────┘
         └─────────────┘           ┌─────────────┐
         ┌─────────────┐           │  Cashiering │
         │   Payroll   │           │    8251     │
         │ accounting  │           └─────────────┘
         │    8214     │           ┌─────────────┐
         └─────────────┘           │  Credit and │
         ┌─────────────┐           │ collections │
         │  Accounts   │           │    8261     │
         │   payable   │           └─────────────┘
         │    8215     │
         └─────────────┘
         ┌─────────────┐
         │  Plant and  │
         │  equipment  │
         │    8216     │
         └─────────────┘
         ┌─────────────┐
         │  Inventory  │
         │ accounting  │
         │    8217     │
         └─────────────┘
         ┌─────────────┐
         │    Data     │
         │ processing  │
         │    8231     │
         └─────────────┘
```

record. Some advocate recording the replacement cost of capital assets, while others recommend using the amount paid for the asset plus operating expenses. The cost value concept has been found to be most appropriate and reasonable because it requires that something of value, that is, cash, be exchanged for an item or service in order for the transaction to be entered in the accounting system. Certainly, an important advantage of using the cost of an item or service is that well-documented proof that the transaction actually occurred can be obtained.

Journals and Ledgers

Seawell differentiates between accounting journals and ledgers in this manner:[8]

> journal: a book of original entry wherein transactions are recorded in chronological sequence.
> ledger: the groups of accounts used in recording the transactions of the hospital—a book of secondary entry.

The hospital's journal system might include such journals as the:

- General Journal
- Cash Receipts
- Cash Disbursements
- Purchase
- Revenue

Basically, journals are books of original entry, while ledgers are support documents. Ledgers can include the:

- General Ledger
- Patient Accounts Receivable
- Plant Equipment and Depreciation
- Payroll
- Inventory
- Accounts Payable

Historically, hospital accounting journals were maintained manually on columnar paper sheets bound together in "post binders." Ledgers were maintained on hard sheets of paper and stored in filing trays. With the advent of automated data processing, journals and ledgers are printed and maintained by computer and stored according to the user's needs.

THE ACCOUNTING PROCESS

The accounting process consists of the systems and procedures required for recording and maintaining the accounting transactions during an accounting period—usually not shorter than one month nor longer than one year. Most hospitals end each accounting period at the end of each month and develop annual statements based upon the operations of 12 months. An annual accounting period, usually called a fiscal year, need not begin on January 1 and end on December 31. Furthermore, there is an accounting system that divides a year into 13 accounting periods of identical length, that is, four weeks. This system eliminates the need to adjust accrual journal entries, for example, payroll, for the odd number of days in a month.

The accounting process, as illustrated in Figure 3–2, begins with source documentation for services rendered to patients, services or items purchased for the hospital, and cash received or disbursed by the hospital. The process ends with the development of four principal financial statements:

1. balance sheet
2. revenue and expense statement
3. cash flow statement
4. statement of changes in financial position

It is important to understand that all the information from the journals is merged into the general ledger from which the financial statements are generated.

In the accounting process, each asset, liability, equity, revenue, and expense account in the hospital's chart of accounts has a separate ledger card or record on which each debit and credit transaction affecting both the account and the balance of the account are identified. Together, all these ledger accounts are referred to as the hospital's general ledger.

Balance Sheet

The balance sheet, which is occasionally referred to as the statement of financial position or the statement of condition, shows the financial position, that is, assets, liabilities, and equity, of the hospital at a specific time, namely, when the accounting records are closed at the end of the accounting

Figure 3-2 The Accounting Process

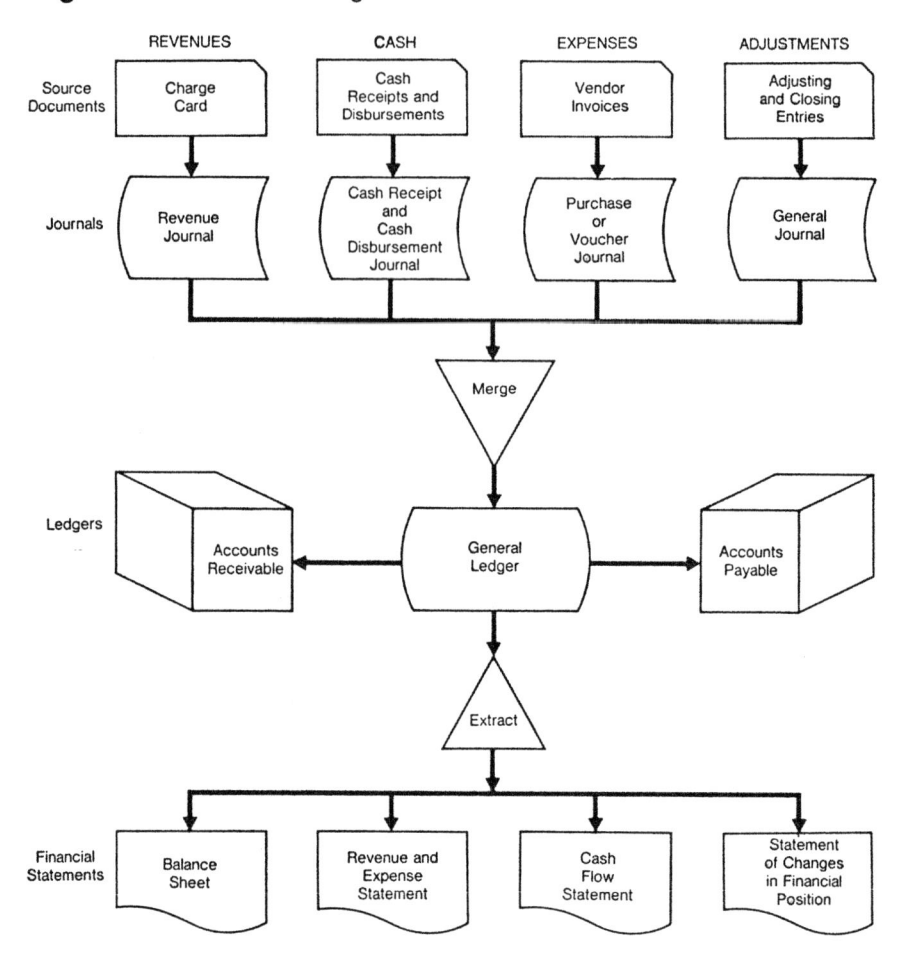

period. The hospital's financial position will change as soon as the hospital incurs an additional expense such as wages or supplies, or renders a service through a revenue department. The formula for the balance sheet is:

Assets = Liabilities + Equity

The hospital's equity is the difference between the hospital's total assets and its total liabilities. Equity has many synonyms, for example:

- capital
- net worth
- surplus
- retained earnings
- fund balance
- stockholders' equity
- owners' equity

In reality, equity, or any other term used in its place, represents the hospital's net assets.

Revenue and Expense Statement

The revenue and expense statement, which has several other titles such as statement of operations, income statement, or profit and loss statement, reports all the hospital's operating and nonoperating revenue as well as the expenses it has incurred during the accounting period and shows the net profit (or loss) for the accounting or operating period. The formulas for the revenue and expense statement are:

- Revenue = Expense + Profit (or Loss)
- Profit (or Loss) = Revenue − Expenses

The basic distinction between the balance sheet and the revenue and expense statement is time. The balance sheet represents the hospital's financial position or condition at *one* specific point in time; the revenue and expense statement reflects the results of revenue and expense transactions *over a period of time*.

Cash Flow Statement

The cash flow statement is a supplemental or analytical statement that identifies either actual or projected cash receipts (inflows) and cash disbursements (outflows) for a period of time. The cash flow statement can be developed for any period of time desired by management. For example, cash flow can be reported on a daily, weekly, monthly, annual, or long-range basis.

Exhibit 3–2 is an example of a combination daily/monthly cash report. It starts with a beginning cash balance, which represents the cash on hand at the beginning of the period, and ends with the cash balance as of the day of the report. Tables 3–5 and 3–6 illustrate cash flow projections for a one-year period and a four-year period, respectively, based on income and expense summaries in Tables 3–7 and 3–8. In the one-year cash flow projection, cash is reported on a monthly basis, while the four-year cash flow forecast shows cash by quarter during the first year and in total annual amounts for the subsequent years.

Exhibit 3–2 Daily Cash Flow Analysis Form

Memorial Hospital, Anytown, U.S.A.
Daily Cash Flow Analysis
For the Month of _____ 19___

Date: _____ 19___

	Today	Month-to-Date
Beginning Cash Balance	$ _____	$ _____
Cash Inflows		
Accounts Receivable	$ _____	$ _____
Borrowings	_____	_____
Other (specify) _____	_____	_____
Total Cash Inflows	$ _____	$ _____
Total Cash on Hand	$ _____	$ _____
Cash Outflows		
Payroll	$ _____	$ _____
Accounts Payable	_____	_____
Long-term Liabilities	_____	_____
Other (specify) _____	_____	_____
Total Cash Outflows	$ _____	$ _____
Ending Cash Balance		

Table 3-5 One-Year Cash Flow Projection, Memorial Hospital, Anytown, U.S.A.

Year One

	1 Sept.	2 Oct.	3 Nov.	4 Dec.	5 Jan.	6 Feb.	7 Mar.	8 Apr.	9 May	10 June	11 July	12 Aug.	Total
Beginning Cash Balance	$ - 0 -	$ 23	$ 838	$ 653	$ 844	$ 473	$ 102	$ 775	$ 10	$ 41	$ 217	$ 166	$ - 0 -
Cash Inflows:													
Accounts receivable	$ - 0 -	$ - 0 -	$ - 0 -	$ - 0 -	$ - 0 -	$ - 0 -	$ 3,534	$ 7,980	$14,136	$17,100	$24,738	$30,780	$ 98,268
Borrowings/Investments	12,000	75,000	18,000	27,000	36,000	29,000	27,000	30,000	33,000	29,000	22,000	28,000	366,000
Total cash inflows	$12,000	$75,000	$18,000	$27,000	$36,000	$29,000	$30,534	$37,980	$47,136	$46,100	$46,738	$58,780	$464,268
Cash on Hand	$12,000	$75,023	$18,838	$27,653	$36,844	$29,473	$30,636	$38,755	$47,146	$46,141	$46,955	$58,946	$464,268
Cash Outflows:													
Corporate payroll and benefits	$11,977	$17,185	$17,185	$17,185	$18,747	$18,747	$18,747	$18,747	$18,747	$24,476	$24,476	$27,288	$233,507
Unit payroll and benefits	- 0 -	- 0 -	- 0 -	7,874	7,874	7,874	7,874	15,748	15,748	15,748	15,748	23,622	118,110
Physicians	- 0 -	- 0 -	- 0 -	750	750	750	1,240	2,250	2,610	2,700	3,565	4,780	19,395
Corporate accounts payable	- 0 -	57,000	1,000	1,000	1,000	1,000	1,000	1,000	1,000	1,000	1,000	1,000	67,000
Unit accounts payable	- 0 -	- 0 -	- 0 -	- 0 -	8,000	1,000	1,000	1,000	9,000	2,000	2,000	2,000	26,000
Total cash outflows	$11,977	$74,185	$18,185	$26,809	$36,371	$29,371	$29,861	$38,745	$47,105	$45,924	$46,789	$58,690	$464,012
Ending Cash Balance	$ 23	$ 838	$ 653	$ 844	$ 473	$ 102	$ 775	$ 10	$ 41	$ 217	$ 166	$ 256	$ 256

Table 3-6 Four-Year Cash Flow Forecast, Memorial Hospital, Anytown, U.S.A.

	Year One				Total			
	1st. Qt.	2nd. Qt.	3rd. Qt.	4th. Qt.	Year One	Year Two	Year Three	Year Four
Beginning Cash Balance	$ - 0 -	$ 653	$ 102	$ 41	$ - 0 -	$ 256	$ 159	$ 19
Cash Inflows:								
Accounts receivable	$ - 0 -	$ - 0 -	$ 25,650	$ 72,618	$ 98,268	$ 948,081	$2,168,394	$3,287,416
Borrowings/Investments	105,000	92,000	90,000	79,000	366,000	70,000	(436,000)	- 0 -
Total cash inflows	$105,000	$ 92,000	$115,650	$151,618	$464,268	$1,018,081	$1,732,394	$3,287,416
Cash on Hand	$105,000	$ 92,653	$115,752	$151,659	$464,268	$1,018,337	$1,732,553	$3,287,416
Cash Outflows:								
Corporate payroll and benefits	$ 46,347	$ 54,679	$ 56,241	$ 76,240	$233,507	$ 388,494	$ 416,196	$ 416,196
Unit payroll and benefits	- 0 -							
Physicians	- 0 -							
Corporate accounts payable	58,000	3,000	3,000	3,000	67,000	12,000	57,500	58,000
Unit accounts payable	- 0 -	9,000	11,000	6,000	26,000	56,000	105,000	164,000
Investment accounts	- 0 -	- 0 -	- 0 -	- 0 -	- 0 -	- 0 -	97,000	1,313,000
Total cash outflows	$104,347	$ 92,551	$115,711	$151,403	$464,012	$1,013,178	$1,732,534	$3,286,529
Ending Cash Balance	$ 653	$ 102	$ 41	$ 256	$ 256	$ 159	$ 19	$ 906

Table 3-7 One-Year Income and Expense Summary, Memorial Hospital, Anytown, U.S.A.

Year One	1 Sept.	2 Oct.	3 Nov.	4 Dec.	5 Jan.	6 Feb.	7 Mar.	8 Apr.	9 May	10 June	11 July	12 Aug.	Total
Volume:													
Calendar days	30	31	30	31	31	28	31	30	31	30	31	31	365
Units	0	0	0	0	1	1	1	1	2	2	2	2	2
Beds	0	0	0	0	18	18	18	18	36	36	36	36	36
Capacity	0	0	0	0	558	504	558	540	1,116	1,080	1,116	1,116	6,030
Patient days	0	0	0	0	62	140	248	300	434	540	713	806	3,243
Percent occupancy	0	0	0	0	11.1	27.8	44.4	55.6	38.9	50.0	63.9	72.2	53.8
Revenue:													
Gross charges	$ - 0 -	$ - 0 -	$ - 0 -	$ - 0 -	$ 3,534	$ 7,980	$14,136	$17,100	$24,738	$30,780	$40,641	$45,942	$184,851
Expense:													
Corporate:													
Staff and benefits	$11,977	$17,185	$17,185	$17,185	$18,747	$18,747	$18,747	$18,747	$18,747	$24,476	$24,476	$27,288	$233,507
Public relations	55,000	- 0 -	- 0 -	- 0 -	- 0 -	- 0 -	- 0 -	- 0 -	- 0 -	- 0 -	- 0 -	- 0 -	55,000
Miscellaneous expenses	2,000	1,000	1,000	1,000	1,000	1,000	1,000	1,000	1,000	1,000	1,000	1,000	13,000
Total corporate expenses	$68,977	$18,185	$18,185	$18,185	$19,747	$19,747	$19,747	$19,747	$19,747	$25,476	$25,476	$28,288	$301,507
Units:													
Staff and benefits	$ - 0 -	$ - 0 -	$ - 0 -	$ 7,874	$ 7,874	$ 7,874	$ 7,874	$15,748	$15,748	$15,748	$15,748	$23,622	$118,110
Physicians	- 0 -	- 0 -	- 0 -	750	750	750	1,240	2,250	2,610	2,700	3,565	4,780	19,395
Training and travel	- 0 -	- 0 -	- 0 -	8,000	- 0 -	- 0 -	- 0 -	8,000	- 0 -	- 0 -	- 0 -	8,000	24,000
Miscellaneous expenses	- 0 -	- 0 -	- 0 -	- 0 -	1,000	1,000	1,000	1,000	2,000	2,000	2,000	2,000	12,000
Total units expenses	$ - 0 -	$ - 0 -	$ - 0 -	$16,624	$ 9,624	$ 9,624	$10,114	$26,998	$20,358	$20,448	$21,313	$38,402	$173,505
Total Expense	$68,977	$18,185	$18,185	$34,809	$29,371	$29,371	$29,861	$46,745	$40,105	$45,924	$46,789	$66,690	$475,012
Profit (Loss)	($68,977)	($18,185)	($18,185)	($34,809)	($25,837)	($21,391)	($15,725)	($29,645)	($15,367)	($15,144)	($6,148)	($20,748)	($290,161)

The Hospital Accounting Process 45

Table 3–8 Four-Year Income and Expense Summary, Memorial Hospital, Anytown, U.S.A.

	Year One					Total			
	1st. Qt.	2nd. Qt.	3rd. Qt.	4th. Qt.	Year One	Year Two	Year Three	Year Four	
Volume:									
Calendar days	91	90	92	92	365	365	365	365	
Units	- 0 -	1	2	2	2	6	11	11	
Beds	- 0 -	18	36	36	36	108	198	198	
Capacity	- 0 -	1,062	2,214	3,312	6,030	29,610	56,448*	72,270*	
Patient days	- 0 -	202	982	2,059	3,243	20,043	41,824	59,193	
Percent occupancy	- 0 -	19.0	44.3	62.1	53.8	67.7	74.0	81.9	
Revenue:									
Gross charges	$ - 0 -	$ 11,514	$ 55,974	$117,363	$184,851	$1,142,451	$2,383,968	$3,374,001	
Expense:									
Corporate:									
Staff and benefits	$ 46,347	$ 54,679	$ 56,241	$ 76,240	$233,507	$ 388,494	$ 416,196	$ 416,196	
Public relations	55,000	- 0 -	- 0 -	- 0 -	55,000	- 0 -	40,000	40,000	
Miscellaneous expenses	4,000	3,000	3,000	3,000	13,000	12,000	18,000	18,000	
Total corporate expenses	$105,347	$ 57,679	$ 59,241	$ 79,240	$301,507	$ 400,494	$ 474,196	$ 474,196	
Units:									
Staff and benefits	$ - 0 -	$ 23,622	$ 39,370	$ 55,118	$118,110	$ 456,692	$ 842,518	$1,039,368	
Physicians	- 0 -	2,250	6,100	11,045	19,395	104,992	214,320	295,965	
Training and travel	- 0 -	8,000	8,000	8,000	24,000	32,000	32,000	32,000	
Miscellaneous expenses	- 0 -	2,000	4,000	6,000	12,000	51,000	103,000	132,000	
Total units expenses	$ - 0 -	$ 35,872	$ 57,470	$ 80,163	$173,505	$ 644,684	$1,191,838	$1,499,333	
Total Expense	$105,347	$ 93,551	$116,711	$159,403	$475,012	$1,045,178	$1,666,034	$1,973,529	
Profit (Loss), before taxes	($105,347)	($ 82,037)	($ 60,737)	($ 42,040)	($290,161)	$ 97,273	$ 717,934	$1,400,472	
Percent of profit to revenue					(156.9)	8.5	30.1	41.5	

* Capacity differs due to scheduling of unit openings.

The Hospital Accounting Process 47

It is imperative for a hospital's financial viability not only to maintain daily and monthly cash flow reports, but also to develop and maintain a long-range cash report, that is, one that shows cash flow projections for one to three years. These reports are especially essential because of all the changing reimbursement regulations imposed by third party payers such as Medicare and Medicaid.

The patient account manager should play a key role in the cash flow reporting and analysis process because accounts receivable is the largest single source of cash flow from hospital operations. In addition, the patient account manager should participate in the process to give the cash flow analysis greater creditability and to ensure his/her self-development and professional survival.

Statement of Changes in Financial Position

The statement of changes in financial position is a comprehensive financial statement that identifies all the changes that have occurred from one balance sheet period to the next. This statement is sometimes referred to as the statement of sources and application of funds; differences in liability accounts reflect the sources of funds, and changes in asset values are classified as applications of funds. The statement of changes in financial position in Table 3–9 was developed using the two balance sheet period changes as reported in the comparative balance sheet in Table 3–10. The statement includes a subsection entitled "Changes in Working Capital" totaling $25,000 which is tied into the "Funds Applied" section.

Working Capital

Working capital has a variety of definitions depending on one's interpretation of the term and its related purpose. For example, a businessperson or an economist may consider the current assets of a business to be working capital. In this book, working capital means the difference between a hospital's total current assets and its total current liabilities:

Working Capital = Current Assets − Current Liabilities

Working capital could be called net current assets. A number of factors affect the working capital requirements of a hospital. An appraisal of these requirements can guide management in estimating the need for future corrective measures. For example, Table 3–9 shows that $120,000 was needed to finance the increase in patient accounts receivable. Assuming net average daily charges to patients of $8,700 in 19x1 and $9,000 in 19x2,

Table 3–9 Statement of Changes in Financial Position

Memorial Hospital, Anytown, U.S.A.
Statement of Changes in Financial Position
From December 31, 19x1 to December 31, 19x2

Funds Provided by:	
Net Operating Profit	$240,000
Depreciation	100,000
Total Funds Provided from Operations	$340,000
Funds Applied to:	
Purchase of Plant and Equipment	$250,000
Reduction of Mortgage Payable	65,000
Increase in Working Capital (see below)	25,000
Total Funds Applied	$340,000
Changes in Working Capital	
Increases (Decreases) in Current Assets:	
Patient Accounts Receivable	$120,000
Inventories	(5,000)
Prepaid Expenses	5,000
Net Increase in Current Assets	$120,000
Increases (Decreases) in Current Liabilities:	
Accounts Payable	$ 10,000
Payroll Taxes Payable	(5,000)
Short-term Notes Payable	90,000
Net Increase in Current Liabilities	$ 95,000
Increase in Working Capital	$ 25,000

this would mean an increase of 10.6 days in the number of days of average daily charges uncollected (see summary in Table 3–11).

Further, assuming that the hospital could invest the $120,000 at 12 percent, the opportunity costs (which will be discussed in Chapter 4) to the hospital would be $14,000 per year. To put it another way, if the hospital had to borrow the $120,000 in the open market to finance its patient accounts receivable at 18 percent, the additional annual cost would be $21,600.

APPLICATION OF THE ACCOUNTING PROCESS

To illustrate the mechanics of the hospital accounting process and the development of a hospital's financial statements, we will assume that during June 19x1, a group of investors purchased the assets of Memorial Hospital

Table 3-10 Comparative Balance Sheet

Memorial Hospital, Anytown, U.S.A.
Comparative Balance Sheet
As of December 31, 19x1 and 19x2

	19x1	19x2	Increase (Decrease)
Assets			
Cash on Hand	$ 40,000	$ 40,000	$ - 0 -
Short-term Investments	30,000	30,000	- 0 -
Net Patient Accounts Receivable	700,000	820,000	120,000
Inventories	50,000	45,000	(5,000)
Prepaid Expenses	25,000	30,000	5,000
Total Current Assets	$ 845,000	$ 965,000	$120,000
Land, Plant, and Equipment	6,000,000	6,250,000	250,000
Less Accumulative Depreciation	1,250,000	1,350,000	100,000 (B)
Net Land, Plant, and Equipment	$4,750,000	$4,900,000	$150,000
Total Assets	$5,595,000	$5,865,000	$270,000
Liabilities			
Accounts Payable	$ 60,000	$ 70,000	$ 10,000
Payroll Taxes Payable	55,000	50,000	(5,000)
Short-term Notes Payable	75,000	165,000	90,000
Total Current Liabilities	$ 190,000	$ 285,000	$ 95,000
Mortgage Payable	3,510,000	3,445,000	(65,000)
Total Liabilities	$3,700,000	$3,730,000	$ 30,000
Net Worth	1,895,000	2,135,000	240,000 (A)
Total Liabilities and Net Worth	$5,595,000	$5,865,000	$270,000

(A) Net Operating Profit for 19x2 = $240,000
(B) Provision for Depreciation during 19x2 = $100,000

---

of Anytown, U.S.A., for $7,500,000, paying $3,000,000 in cash and financing the balance with a long-term ten percent mortgage.

The accounting transactions the hospital incurred during the month of June 19x1 are recorded initially in the journal as follows:

1. Plant Assets.. $7,500,000
    Owners' Equity $3,000,000
    Mortgage Payable 4,500,000
    To record the purchase of Memorial Hospital as of June 1, 19x1.

Table 3-11 Ratio Analysis of Patient Accounts Receivable

Memorial Hospital, Anytown, U.S.A.
Ratio Analysis of Patient Accounts Receivable
As of December 31, 19x2

Days Uncollected	19x1	19x2
Net average daily charges to patients	$ 8,700	$ 9,000
Net patient accounts receivable	700,000	820,000
Number of days of average daily charge uncollected	80.5	91.1

2. Accounts Receivable $1,500,000
   Routine Services Revenue $900,000
   Ancillary Services Revenue.................... 600,000
   To record the patient revenue for the month of June 19x1 from the Revenue Journal.
3. Inventory $250,000
   Accounts Payable............................... $250,000
   To record the supplies purchased and inventoried during the month of June 19x1 from the Purchase Journal.
4. Salary Expense.................................. $850,000
   Cash... $800,000
   Payroll Taxes Payable......................... 50,000
   To record the payroll expenses paid and payable for the month of June 19x1 from the Payroll Journal.
5. Cash... $1,200,000
   Accounts Receivable $1,200,000
   To record the cash received during the month of June 19x1 from the Cash Receipts Journal.
6. Depreciation $70,000
   Reserve for Depreciation....................... $70,000
   To record the provision for depreciation expense for the month of June 19x1 from the Plant Journal.
7. Interest Expense.................................. $37,500
   Mortgage Payable 20,000
   Cash... $57,500
   To record the mortgage payment and interest expense for the month of June 19x1 from the Cash Disbursements Journal.

8. Provision for Bad Debts........................... $75,000
   Reserve for Bad Debts and Allowances...................... $75,000

   To record the provision for bad debts at the rate of five percent of gross patient revenue for the month of June 19x1 from the General Journal.

9. Accounts Payable................................. $200,000
   Cash... $200,000

   To record the amount paid on accounts payable during the month of June 19x1 from the Cash Disbursements Journal.

10. Provision for Contractual Allowances $90,000
    Reserve for Bad Debts and Allowances...................... $90,000

    To record the provision for contractual allowances (Medicare, Blue Cross, and Medicaid) for the month of June 19x1 from the General Journal.

11. Prepaid Expenses................................. $42,500
    Cash... $42,500

    To record the payment of the hospital's annual insurance premiums from the Cash Disbursements Journal.

12. Insurance Expense $3,500
    Prepaid Expenses.. $3,500

    To record the provision for insurance expense for the month of June 19x1 from the General Journal.

13. Supply Expense $200,000
    Inventory $200,000

    To record the supplies requisitioned during the month of June 19x1 from the Inventory Journal.

14. Short-term Investments $90,000
    Cash... $90,000

    To record the cash invested in short-term notes during the month of June 19x1 from the Cash Disbursements Journal.

52   PATIENT ACCOUNT MANAGEMENT

15. Provision for Income Taxes...................... $87,000
    Income Taxes Payable $87,000
    To record the provision for income taxes payable from the General Journal.

These transactions are then transferred, or posted, to the general ledger T-account as shown in Table 3–12. After all the posting to the general ledger T-accounts is completed, a balance is computed for each account for the end of the accounting period and summarized in a general ledger trial balance as shown in Table 3–13. Total debits must equal total credits in this analysis regardless of the financial statement in which these accounts will ultimately appear.

As a general rule, accounts are listed in the general ledger trial balance in numerical order corresponding to the chart of accounts. In other words, asset accounts appear first and are followed by liability, equity, revenue, and expense accounts.

The statement of financial position in Table 3–14 was developed using all the asset, liability, and equity accounts; however, the statement of operations in Table 3–15 was developed from only revenue and expense accounts. It is important to note that in order to have the total assets equal the total liabilities and net worth in the statement of financial position, it was necessary to add the net operating profit (or loss) to the hospital's net worth. Thus, to complete the formula:

$$\text{Assets} = \text{Liabilities} + \text{Net Worth}$$
or
$$\$7,754,000 = \$4,667,000 + \$3,087,000$$

The cash flow statement in Table 3–16 was developed from the analysis of the transactions in the T-account activity in the general ledger cash account in Table 3–12, page 53. The ending cash balance of $10,000 also appears as a current asset in the hospital's statement of financial position. In this example, the investors purchased only the fixed plant assets and not the other assets and liabilities; therefore, no statement of changes in financial position was developed.

In this book, the term "statement of financial position" is preferred to "balance sheet" because the former term more accurately describes what the statement really is—the presentation of the financial position of the hospital at one point in time. Also the term "statement of operations" is preferred to "income and expense statement" because the first term more accurately indicates the actual information the statement contains—the net

Table 3-12 General Ledger T-Account

Memorial Hospital, Anytown, U.S.A.
General Ledger T-Account

Cash		Accounts Receivable		Reserve for Bad Debts and Allowances	
(5) 1,200,000	(4) 800,000	(2) 1,500,000	(5) 1,200,000		(8) 75,000
	(7) 57,500	Bal. 300,000			(10) 90,000
	(9) 200,000				Bal. 165,000
	(11) 42,500				
	(14) 90,000				
Bal. 10,000					

Prepaid Expenses		Inventory		Short-term Investments	
(11) 42,500	(12) 3,500	(3) 250,000	(13) 200,000	(14) 90,000	
Bal. 39,000		Bal. 50,000		Bal. 90,000	

Plant Assets		Reserve for Depreciation		Accounts Payable	
(1) 7,500,000			(6) 70,000	(9) 200,000	(3) 250,000
Bal. 7,500,000			Bal. 70,000		Bal. 50,000

Payroll Taxes Payable		Income Taxes Payable		Mortgage Payable	
	(4) 50,000	(15) 87,000		(7) 20,000	(1) 4,500,000
	Bal. 50,000				Bal. 4,480,000

Owners' Equity		Routine Services Revenue		Ancillary Services Revenue	
	(1) 3,000,000		(2) 900,000		(2) 600,000
	Bal. 3,000,000				

Provision for Bad Debts		Provision for Contractual Allowances		Salary Expense	
(8) 75,000		(10) 90,000		(4) 850,000	

Table 3–12 continued

Supply Expense	Interest Expense	Insurance Expense
(13) 200,000	(7) 37,500	(12) 3,500

	Depreciation	Provision for Income Taxes
	(6) 70,000	(15) 87,000

Table 3–13 Trial Balance

Memorial Hospital, Anytown, U.S.A.
General Ledger Trial Balance
As of June 30, 19x1

Account	Debits	Credits
Cash	$ 10,000	$
Accounts Receivable	300,000	
Reserve for Bad Debts and Allowances		165,000
Prepaid Expenses	39,000	
Inventory	50,000	
Short-term Investments	90,000	
Plant Assets	7,500,000	
Reserve for Depreciation		70,000
Accounts Payable		50,000
Payroll Taxes Payable		50,000
Income Taxes Payable		87,000
Mortgage Payable		4,480,000
Owners' Equity		3,000,000
Revenue Routine Services		900,000
Revenue Ancillary Services		600,000
Provision for Bad Debts	75,000	
Provision for Contractual Allowances	90,000	
Salary Expense	850,000	
Supply Expense	200,000	
Interest Expense	37,500	
Insurance Expense	3,500	
Depreciation Expense	70,000	
Provision for Income Taxes	87,000	
Total	$9,402,000	$9,402,000

Table 3–14 Statement of Financial Position

Memorial Hospital, Anytown, U.S.A.
Statement of Financial Position
As of June 30, 19x1

ASSETS

Current Assets		
Cash		$ 10,000
Accounts Receivable	$ 300,000	
Less: Reserve for Bad Debts and Allowances	165,000	$ 135,000
Prepaid Expenses		39,000
Inventory		50,000
Short-term Investments		90,000
Total Current Assets		$ 324,000
Plant and Equipment	$7,500,000	
Less: Reserve for Depreciation	70,000	
Net Plant and Equipment		7,430,000
Total Assets		$7,754,000

LIABILITIES AND NET WORTH

Current Liabilities	
Accounts Payable	$ 50,000
Payroll Taxes Payable	50,000
Income Taxes Payable	87,000
Total Current Liabilities	187,000
Mortgage Payable	$4,480,000
Total Liabilities	$4,667,000
Net Worth	$3,000,000
Plus Net Operating Profit (Loss)	87,000
Total Net Worth	$3,087,000
Total Liabilities and Net Worth	$7,754,000

Table 3–15 Statement of Operations

Memorial Hospital, Anytown, U.S.A.
Statement of Operations
For the Month Ending June 30, 19x1

Gross Revenue		
Routine Services		$ 900,000
Ancillary Services		600,000
Total Gross Revenue		$1,500,000
Deductions from Gross Revenue		
Provision for Bad Debts	$ 75,000	
Provision for Contractual Allowances	$ 90,000	
Total Deductions from Gross Revenue		$ 165,000
Net Revenue		$1,335,000
Operating Expense		
Salaries	$850,000	
Supplies	200,000	
Interest	37,500	
Insurance	3,500	
Depreciation	70,000	
Total Operating Expense		$1,161,000
Net Operating Profit (Loss) before Taxes		$ 174,000
Provision for Income Taxes		$ 87,000
Net Operating Profit (Loss) after Taxes		$ 87,000

results, that is, revenue and expense and profit or loss, of the hospital's operations over a period of time.

In addition, plant assets are included in the operating or general fund rather than establishing a separate plant fund because it is not necessary to use fund accounting if accounting funds are consolidated into one general fund and appropriate asset and reserve accounts are maintained.

In conclusion, the transactions presented in this illustration have been individualized so the reader can interpret and analyze each transaction in terms of its own logic, regardless of the source journal. Balances are identified in the asset, liability, and equity accounts because there are multiple entries in most of the accounts. These accounts are never "closed out"; balances are always brought forward for new accounting periods. Balances in the revenue and expense accounts are not singled out for identification because there is only one entry in each of these accounts. These accounts are always "closed out" at the end of each accounting period.

Table 3–16 Cash Flow Statement

Memorial Hospital, Anytown, U.S.A.
Cash Flow Statement
For the Month of June 19X1

Beginning Cash Balance		$ - 0 -
Cash Inflows		
Accounts Receivable		$1,200,000
Other		- 0 -
Total Cash Inflows		$1,200,000
Total Cash on Hand		$1,200,000
Cash Outflows		
Operating Expenses:		
Payroll	$800,000	
Interest	37,500	
Total Operating Expenses		$ 837,500
Current Assets:		
Prepaid Insurance	$ 42,500	
Short-term Investments	90,000	
Total Current Assets		$ 132,500
Accounts Payable		$ 200,000
Payment on Mortgage		$ 20,000
Total Cash Outflow		$1,190,000
Ending Cash Balance		$ 10,000

NOTES

1. L. Vann Seawell, *Hospital Financial Accounting Theory and Practice* (Chicago: Hospital Financial Management Association, 1975), p. 23.
2. *Annual Hospital Report* (Washington, D.C.: U.S. Department of Health, Education and Welfare, Health Care Financing Administration, February 20, 1980), pp. 3–12 and 3–13.
3. Allen G. Herkimer, Jr., *Understanding Hospital Financial Management* (Germantown, Md.: Aspen Systems Corp., 1978), pp. 24–25.
4. *Chart of Accounts for Hospitals* (Chicago: Department of Health and Human Resources, Health Care Financing Administration, 1973), p. 15.
5. *Annual Hospital Report*, p. 0.2.
6. Ibid., p. 0.3.
7. *Chart of Accounts for Hospitals*, pp. 87–91.
8. Seawell, *Hospital Financial Accounting Theory and Practice*, p. 553.

Chapter 4

Management Accounting and Its Application

The accounting system is the major quantitative information collection, processing, and reporting mechanism in a hospital. An effective hospital accounting system should provide information for the following three purposes:

1. internal reporting to managers for use in planning and controlling current operations
2. internal reporting to managers for use in making special decisions and formulating long-range plans
3. external reporting to third party purchasers of health services, stockholders, governmental agencies, and the community

Horngren states that financial or general accounting has been concerned mainly with the third purpose and has been oriented toward the historical, stewardship aspects of external reporting. He identifies the distinguishing feature of management accounting as its emphasis on the first and second purposes.[1] In fact, most hospitals have been so busy complying with the reporting requirements of outside agencies such as federal and state third party guarantors and trade associations that they have not developed effective internal management information systems.

Both general and management accounting are essential to a hospital's information system. The precise historical information generated by the hospital's general accounting system is the foundation for its management accounting system. General accounting is concerned with basic operating revenues and expenses, while management accounting is concerned with providing all levels of management with information necessary for decision making. A key part of this information is behavior patterns for revenues and expenses under changing conditions. These patterns will be discussed later in this chapter.

MANAGEMENT REPORTING

The key to an effective management accounting and information system is to present data in a way that allows users to receive information they need to know. The key words or phrases in this statement are:

- user
- need to know

The challenge to the patient account manager is to develop, with the cooperation of the accounting and data processing department managers, an information system that will assist in:

- carrying out the patient account department's mission
- analyzing patient accounts receivable timely and accurately
- managing and controlling patient account department expenses
- managing and controlling departmental productivity
- achieving timely and appropriate patient billings

Management accounting and reporting are meant to be working tools for the department's employees as well as its manager. Some patient business services personnel may not be accounting- or numbers-oriented individuals; therefore, management reports should not be limited to columns of numbers. Experience has shown that the best method of designing a management report is for the person responsible for preparing the report to work with its users in designing it. The objective is to communicate in the simplest language possible. The management reporting system should be flexible enough to supply one-time or single-purpose reports as well as routine ones such as monthly reports.

Figures 4–1, 4–2, and 4–3 show how line graphs may be used to represent statistical and financial data and to assist in analyzing trends in key indexes such as:

- gross accounts receivable
- average daily gross charges
- number of days of average gross charges uncollected
- cash flow requirements and projections
- actual cash flow

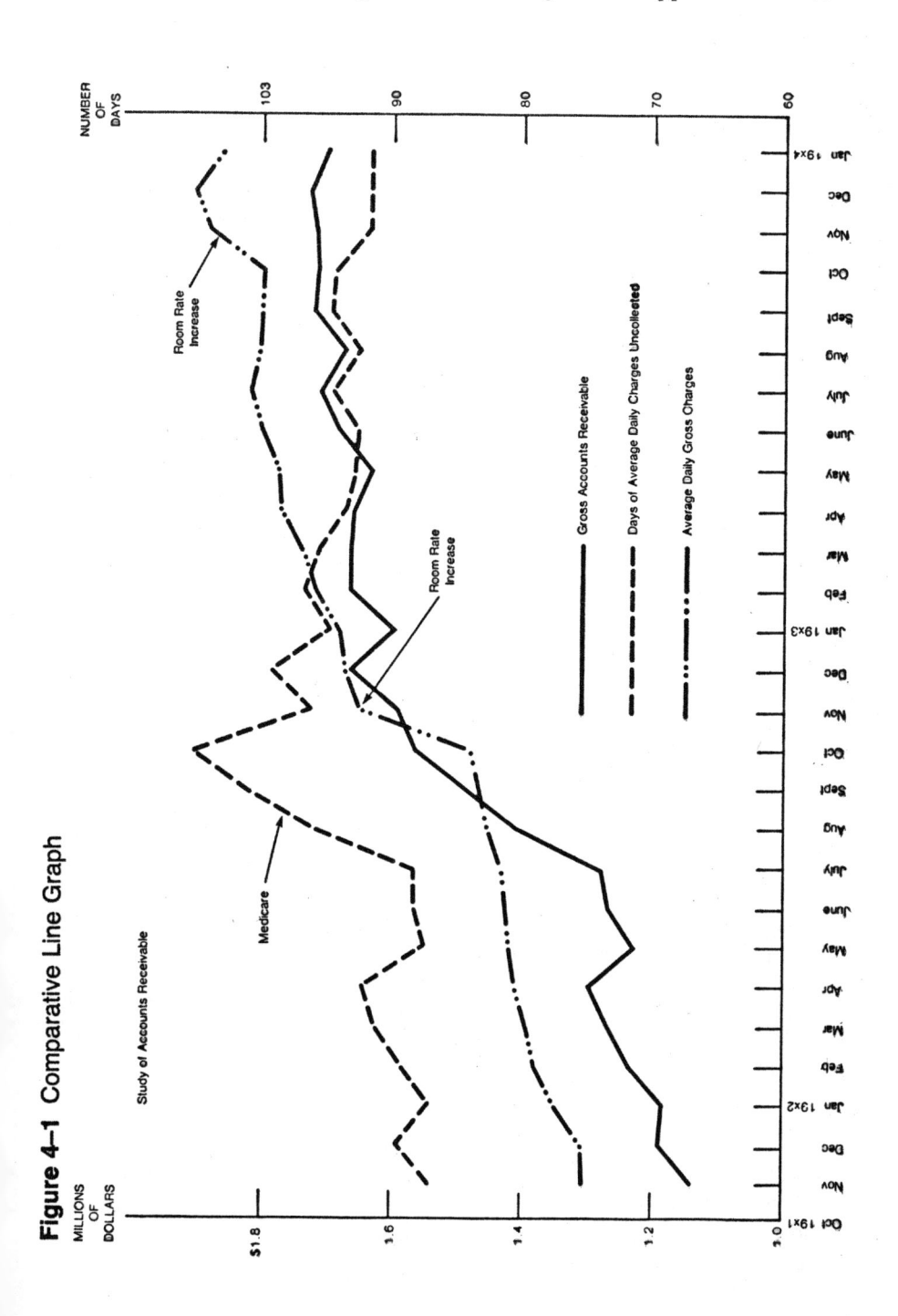

Management Accounting and Its Application 61

Figure 4–1 Comparative Line Graph

Figure 4–2 Flowing Line Graph with Minimum and Maximum

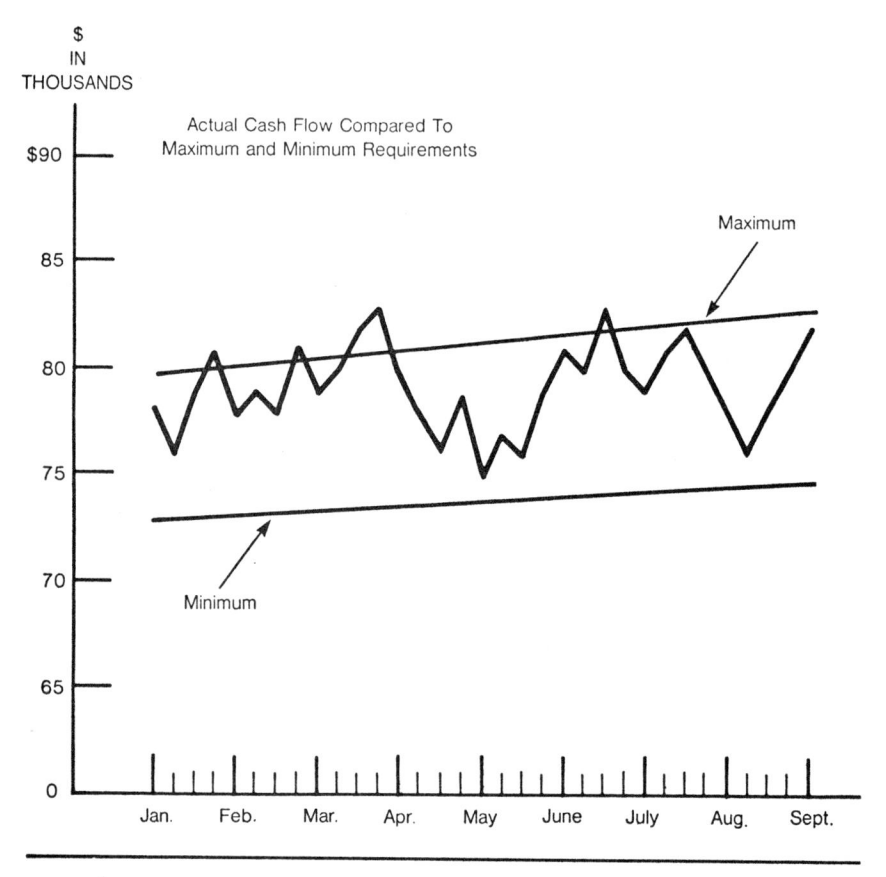

The design of the charts or graphs and the indexes to be depicted in them must be determined by the patient account manager and the users of the information.

PRINCIPLES OF EXPENSE BEHAVIOR

One unique feature of management accounting is that it classifies expenses according to the manner in which they interact under changing conditions. To make effective management decisions, the patient account manager must understand expense characteristics and their behavior as well as their impact on the department and on the total hospital operation.

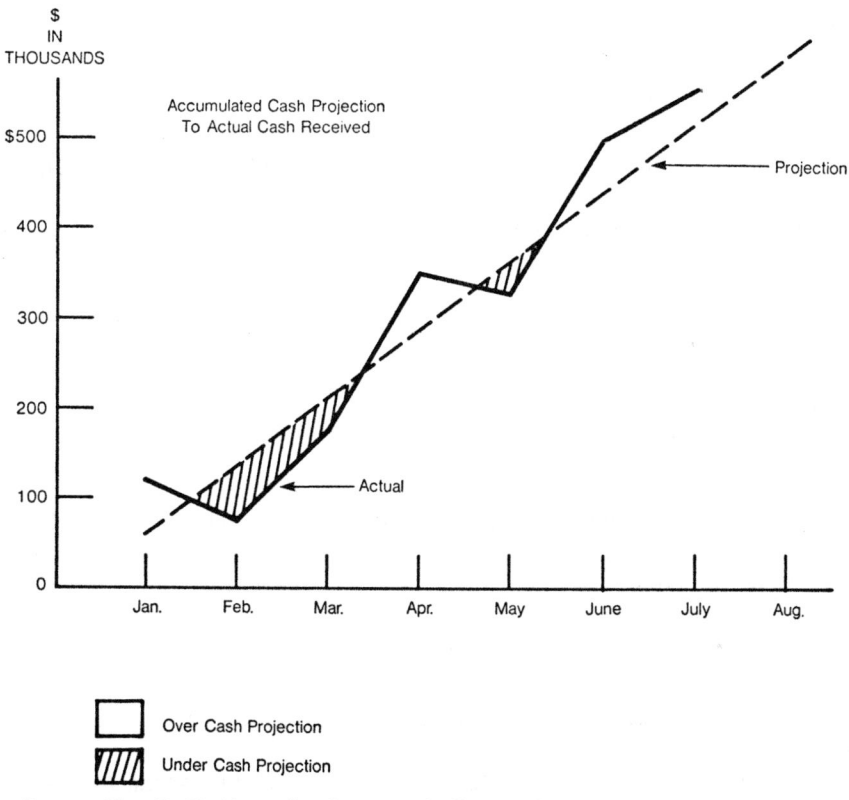

Figure 4–3 Single Shaded Line Graph

Accumulated Cash Projection To Actual Cash Received

☐ Over Cash Projection
▨ Under Cash Projection

Source: Allen G. Herkimer, Jr., *Concepts in Hospital Financial Management*, 2nd ed. (Northridge, Calif.: Alfa Associates, Inc., 1973), pp. 1 and 8.

The expenses with which the patient account manager must be concerned can be divided into three major categories:[2]

1. operating: expenses that are incurred during the normal course of carrying out the day-to-day functions of the department
2. opportunity: expenses (or lost revenue) caused if assets, goods, or services are applied to an alternative use
3. social: expenses that management knowingly or unknowingly imposes on general or specific segments of society as a result of its decisions

Expenses can be classified further as:

- actual
- planned or estimated

Actual costs are expenses that are incurred and can be supported by documentation. Planned or estimated expenses, on the other hand, are those which management predicts through the budgeting process or through other estimates.

Expenses are also categorized as:

- fixed
- variable
- step-variable

Fixed expenses tend to remain relatively constant regardless of volume or amount of work required to produce something (see Figure 4-4). The salary of the patient account manager is an excellent example of a fixed salary expense, and depreciation, liability insurance, and rent are good examples of nonlabor fixed expenses. Fixed expenses can be controlled only before the commitment to expend them, such as a contract, is made.

Figure 4-4 Departmental Fixed Expense, Memorial Hospital, Anytown, U.S.A.

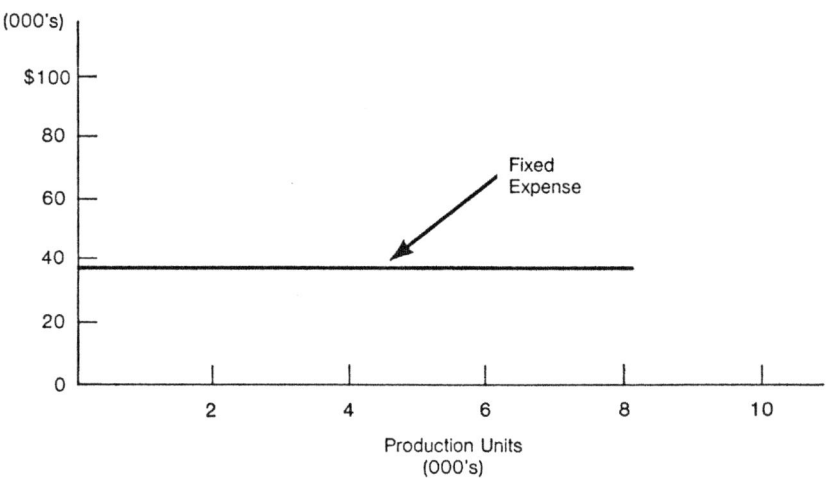

Variable expenses, on the other hand, tend to change in direct relationship to volume or the amount of work produced as shown in Figure 4–5. Billing and admitting forms are examples of variable expenses. Variable expenses can be controlled on a day-to-day basis.

If one consolidates the information in Figures 4–4 and 4–5, one can compute the total costs represented by the fixed and variable expenses. The result is depicted in Figure 4–6. For example, assume that 10,000 units have been produced. The total expense for producing these units would be $10,000. Of that total, fixed expenses represent $4,000, and variable expenses account for $6,000.

The most difficult expense classification to recognize and calculate is the step-variable expense. The behavior of this kind of expense is a combination of the behavior of fixed and variable expenses. A step-variable expense may change abruptly at intervals according to relevant ranges of activity that can be measured in discrete segments. Salaries of billing and admitting clerks and most other nonadministrative personnel tend to be step-variable expenses because a staffing level will usually stay within a relevant range of volume or activity. Most staffing patterns have a certain amount of elasticity; a staff of a given size can handle a suddenly lower volume of activity (negative elasticity) or a suddenly higher volume of activity (positive elasticity). As with variable expenses, step-variable ex-

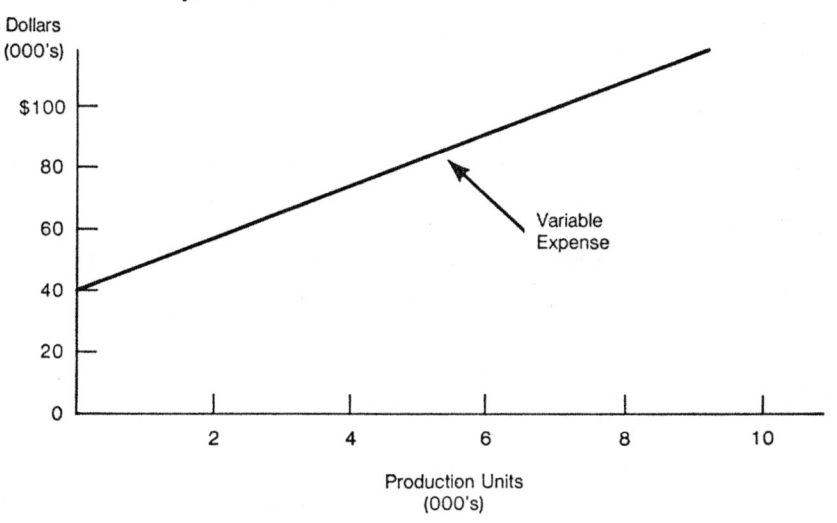

Figure 4–5 Departmental Variable Expense, Memorial Hospital, Anytown, U.S.A.

66   PATIENT ACCOUNT MANAGEMENT

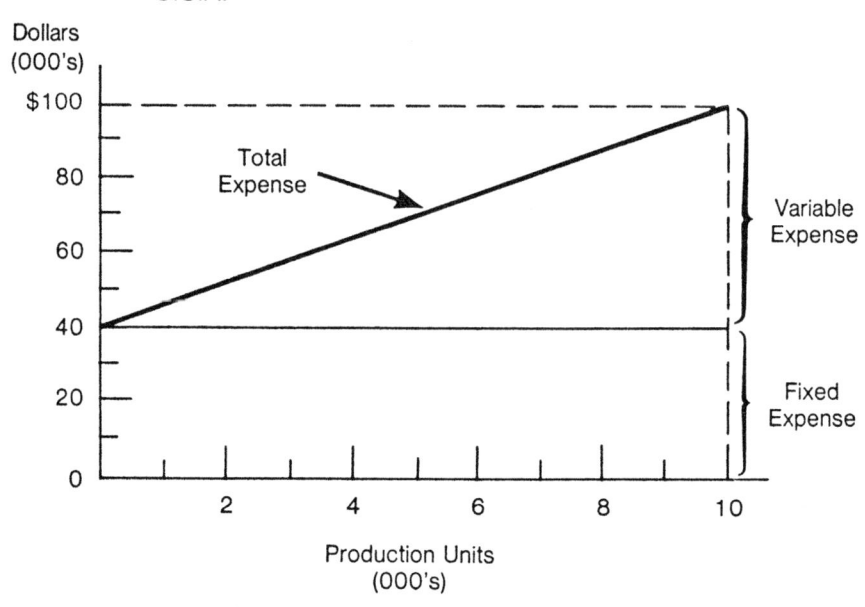

Figure 4–6 Total Departmental Expenses, Memorial Hospital, Anytown, U.S.A.

penses may be controlled on a day-to-day operating basis. Step-variable expenses are controlled by adjusting to trends in workload volume.

For example, suppose that management has determined that three billing clerks can adequately process up to 4,000 bills per billing period. Salaries of the three billing clerks are a step-variable expense because once the billing volume reaches and consistently remains at 5,000, the reasonable elasticity of this staffing pattern has been exceeded, and the staff must be abruptly increased one step (in this case, one billing clerk must be added). Adding one billing clerk automatically establishes a higher range of volume or activity—4,000 to 8,000 bills (as illustrated in Figure 4–7). The new staffing level, four billing clerks, remains fixed as long as billing activity remains within the 4,000 to 8,000 range. When volume reaches 8,000 to 12,000, five and one-half billing clerks will be required. Staffing requirements are based on predetermined production standards, which will be discussed in Chapter 5.

In addition to operating expenses, the patient account manager should consider the impact of his/her decisions on opportunity and social expenses.

Figure 4–7 Step-Variable Staffing Requirements, Memorial Hospital, Anytown, U.S.A.

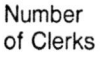

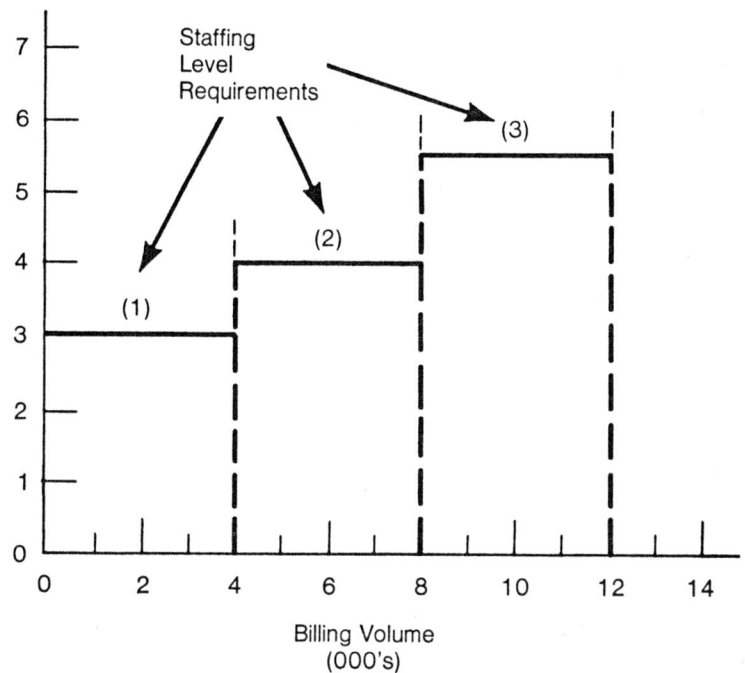

It is necessary to ask questions such as:

- What working capital expense is incurred by the hospital at the present level of uncollected average daily revenue?
- How much are the hospital's service area residents willing to pay for a new, automated billing system?

It is important that each manager realize that almost every decision he or she makes affects not only the hospital's operating expense budget but also the operating expenses of society. For this reason, the patient account manager must weigh all aspects of each decision carefully.

Since the patient account manager is concerned primarily with operating expenses, the balance of this discussion will be directed toward the management of operating expenses. Levels of expense classification are illustrated in Figure 4–8.

Figure 4–8 Levels of Expense Classifications, Memorial Hospital, Anytown, U.S.A.

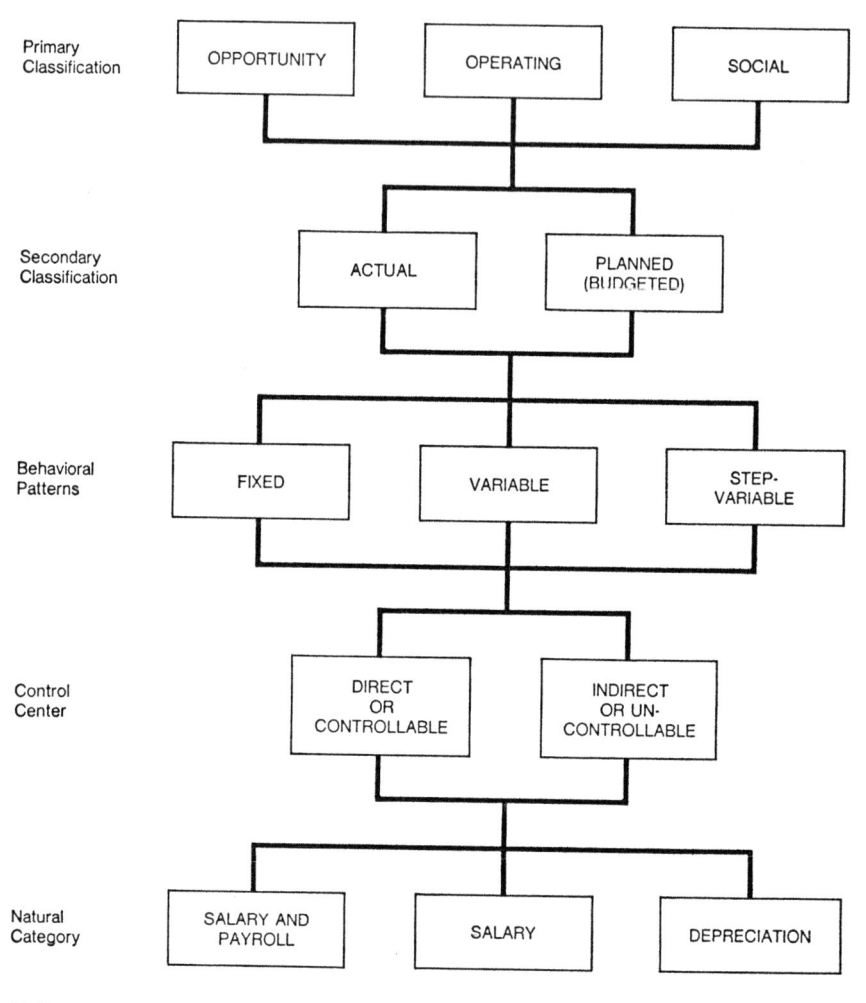

Primary Classification: OPPORTUNITY | OPERATING | SOCIAL

Secondary Classification: ACTUAL | PLANNED (BUDGETED)

Behavioral Patterns: FIXED | VARIABLE | STEP-VARIABLE

Control Center: DIRECT OR CONTROLLABLE | INDIRECT OR UNCONTROLLABLE

Natural Category: SALARY AND PAYROLL | SALARY | DEPRECIATION

Operating expenses are divided into two major categories:

1. direct or controllable: expenses caused by decisions made by the manager and/or subordinates for which they are accountable and responsible
2. indirect or uncontrollable: expenses that are incurred by another supporting department and allocated proportionally to all departments

using such services (for example, number of medical summaries, utilities, repairs, and maintenance)

Operating expenses are divided further into three supplementary classifications:

1. salary and payroll
2. nonsalary
3. depreciation

Salary and payroll expenses, which are caused by a department's staffing pattern, include not only employee salary and wages but also payroll-related fringe benefits such as social security taxes, unemployment taxes, group insurance, and retirement benefits.

This natural expense category is the most significant in the patient business services department because salary and related expenses constitute over 70 percent of the total operating expense in most patient business services departments. Therefore, a key to successful management of the patient business services department is the development and maintenance of staffing patterns based on realistic performance standards.

Nonsalary expenses include all other operating expenses such as office supplies, purchased services, fees, and dues. Depreciation is not included in this expense classification group because it is a noncash expense or provision that represents only a portion of the original cost of a tangible plant asset allocated to a particular accounting period.[3]

OTHER EXPENSE CLASSIFICATIONS

Presently, inflation expense could be the most significant expense in the "other expense" classification with which the patient account manager must contend. Generally, inflation expense is provided for in the budgeting process, but the inflation factor has been highly unpredictable due to general economic conditions. Drucker states that inflation should be considered a genuine expense, adding that there is good reason to adopt, at least internally, a method of accounting in "constant dollars." Drucker concludes that inflation rather than the hospital's performance underlies a good profit.[4]

Replacement expense is the actual or estimated expense of replacing a hospital's present tangible assets. Generally, the term refers to the expense of replacing or renovating a building or office or replacing a piece of equipment such as a computer, typewriter, or desk. Unlike inflation expense, replacement expense can be computed relatively accurately. Replacement expense is not usually recorded as an actual operating expense in the accounting system. However, some hospitals do provide for replacement expense by systematically depositing cash in a special replacement and depreciation investment fund that can be used to replace obsolete assets.

Committed expenses include all fixed expenses that are incurred in the operation of the plant, equipment, and basic or core staff. Examples are depreciation, utilities, taxes, insurance, and salaries for key or core personnel. Committed expenses are sometimes called capacity expenses. As stated earlier, fixed, committed, or capacity expenses can be controlled only before a commitment is made and the contract is signed. Once management has made the decision to buy and has signed a contract, it has passed the "cost control point" and must be content to amortize the expense over a period of time.

Programmed expense is a fixed expense that arises periodically—usually annually—from management decisions that reflect its policies. Examples of programmed expenses include insurance premiums, auditing fees, and training programs. Programmed expenses, as committed expenses, have no relationship to volume or workload and must be controlled before a contract is signed.

To summarize, there are innumerable classifications that can be used to segregate expenses. The degree to which expenses are classified and the terms for these expenses depend on management's need to isolate and control specific expenses. Frequently, management will select key or major expenses—travel in Administration, drugs in Pharmacy, utilities in Plant, or films in Radiology—for closer surveillance and control. The patient account manager must identify his/her own key or major expense items and manage accordingly.

COST ANALYSIS

In analyzing the patient business services department expenses, the total department fixed or capacity expenses, such as billings and admissions, remain constant within a relevant volume range. Total variable department expenses, on the other hand, usually increase in direct proportion to increases in work volume. This phenomenon is illustrated in Figure 4–9.

The following is a cost analysis of the patient business services department's total direct expenses based on the three volume activity points in Figure 4–9.

Figure 4-9 Total Departmental Direct Expenses, Memorial Hospital, Anytown, U.S.A.

Expense Description	Volume Activity Points		
	20-A	60-B	100-C
Fixed Expense	$40,000	$40,000	$40,000
Variable Expense	12,000	36,000	60,000
Total Department Expense	$52,000	$76,000	$100,000

The department's total variable expenses—sixty cents (60¢) per unit of service—are shown in Figure 4-10.

Although the total departmental direct expense curve increases as volume increases, as Figure 4-9 shows, the total production unit cost curve declines as volume increases (see Figure 4-11).

The following is a cost analysis of the patient business services department's total production unit expenses (as shown in Figure 4-11):

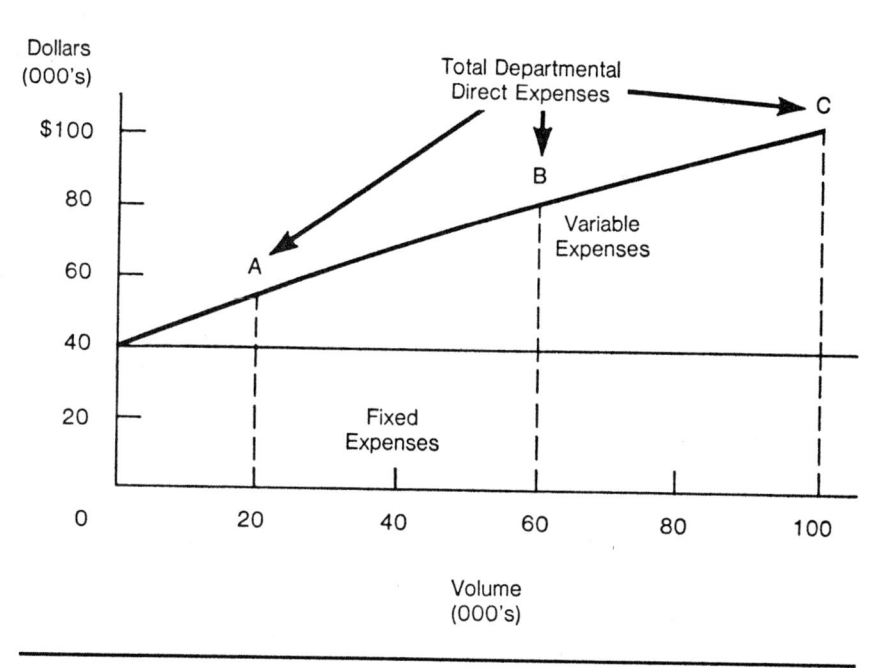

72   PATIENT ACCOUNT MANAGEMENT

Figure 4–10 Total Departmental Direct Variable Expenses, Memorial Hospital, Anytown, U.S.A.

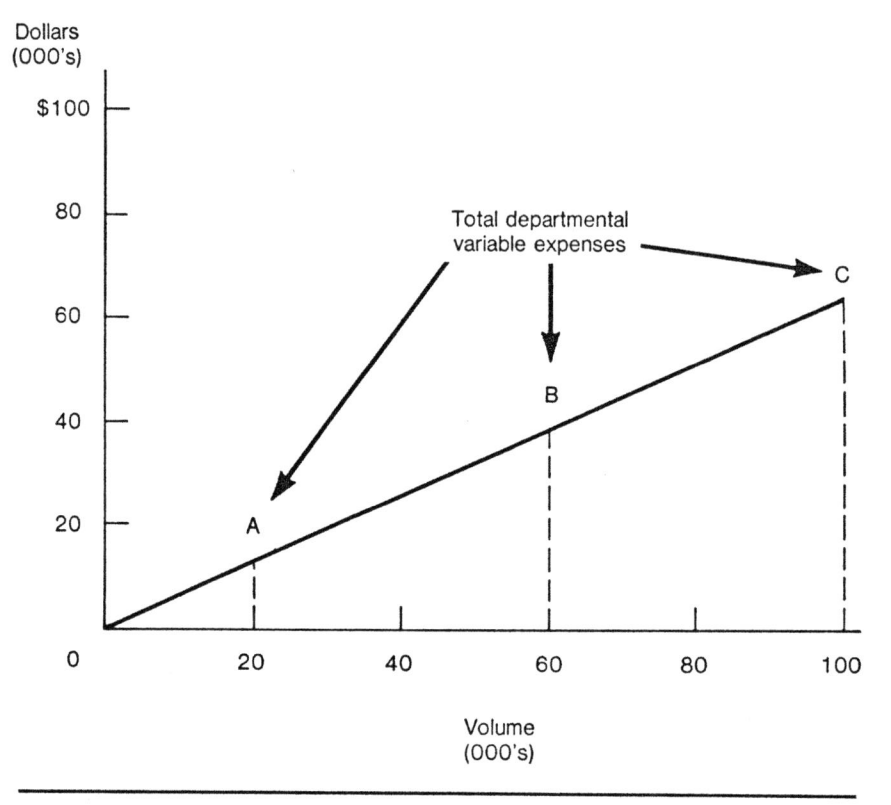

Expense Description	Volume of Billing Activity				
	20,000	40,000	60,000	80,000	100,000
Fixed Expense	$2.00	$1.00	$0.67	$0.50	$0.40
Variable Expense	0.60	0.60	0.60	0.60	0.60
Total Expense Per Production Unit	$2.60	$1.60	$1.27	$1.10	$1.00

Using this analysis, the expense for each billing is $2.60 if the patient business services department produces 20,000 billings, whereas billing unit cost drops to $1.00 when 100,000 billings are produced.

The knowledge of expenses and their related behavior will help the patient account manager control the cost of operating his/her department. Fixed expenses are probably one of the most difficult categories of expenses

Figure 4–11 Total Departmental Production Unit Expenses, Memorial Hospital, Anytown, U.S.A.

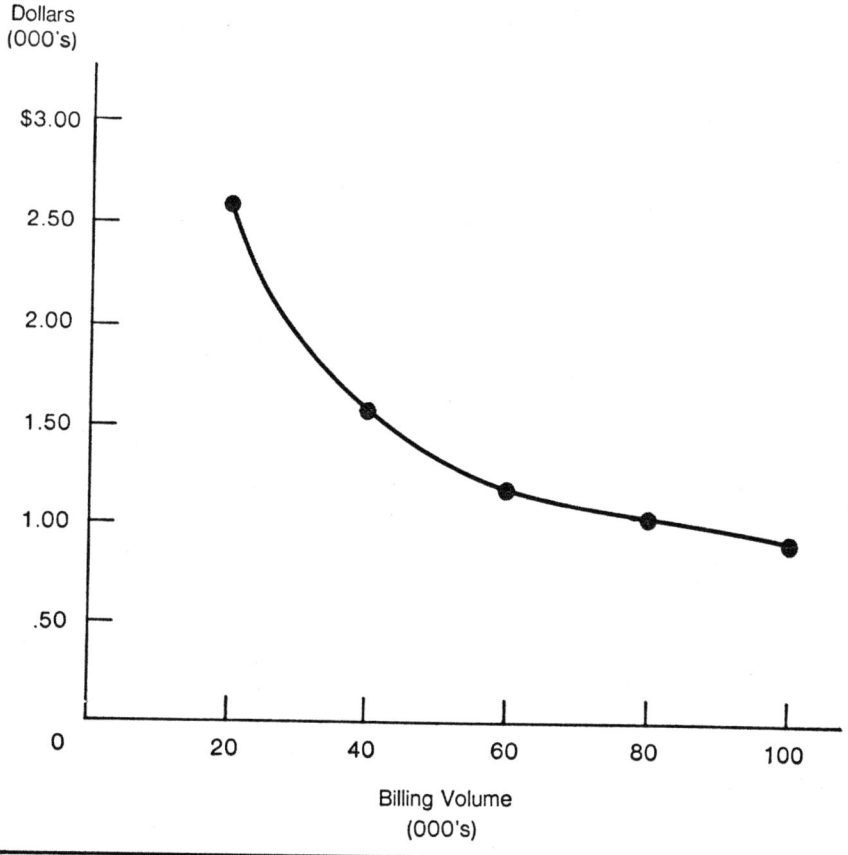

to control, especially after the initial commitment, such as hiring an additional billing clerk, has been made. In such instances, the challenge is to transform the fixed expense into a step-variable or a variable expense to reduce total expenses. That can be accomplished by reducing the number of full-time employees and using more part-time employees or PRNs on an as-needed basis. In general, the key is to control fixed expenses before they are committed and to control variable expenses on a day-to-day operational basis.[5]

APPLICATION OF EXPENSE BEHAVIOR PRINCIPLES

The variable budget is an expense control system that is an excellent application of expense behavior principles. This system uses the standard variable cost concept that establishes a standard rate or expected expense per production unit. The standard rate is computed by dividing the total variable expense by the budgeted or expected total number of units to be produced by the expense category.

To illustrate, assume that the patient account manager has determined that an acceptable and reasonable performance standard per billing clerk is 1,000 bills per month. During the month ending September 30, 19x1, 5,400 bills were processed by six clerks, each earning $1,000 per month. From this information, we extract the following relevant data:

A. Number of full-time clerks	6
B. Monthly performance standard per clerk	1,000 billings
C. Monthly capacity: A × B = C	6,000 billings
D. Monthly salary expense per clerk	$1,000
E. Total monthly salary expense: A × D = E	$6,000
F. Standard salary expense per billing: E ÷ C = F	$1.00

Tables 4–1 and 4–2 illustrate the impact that volume changes and the use of standard expense rates have on a department's productivity and efficiency. In comparing the target budget to actual performance, as shown in Table 4–1, we find no variance in salary expense; however, there is an unfavorable volume variance of 600 billings. Thus, when performance is

Table 4–1 Comparative Analysis of Actual Performance to Target Budget

Memorial Hospital, Anytown, U.S.A.
Patient Business Services Department
Comparative Analysis of Actual Performance to Target Budget
For the Month Ending September 30, 19x1

	Target Budget	Actual Performance	Variance to Budget
Volume (Billings)	6,000	5,400	(600) Unfavorable
Salary Expense	$6,000	$6,000	None

Table 4-2 Comparative Analysis of Actual Performance to Control Budget

Memorial Hospital, Anytown, U.S.A.
Patient Business Services Department
Comparative Analysis of Actual Performance to Control Budget
For the Month Ending September 30, 19x1

	Control Budget	Actual Performance	Variance to Budget
Volume (Billings)	5,400*	5,400	None
Salary Expense	$5,400	$6,000	($600) Unfavorable

* Adjusted to actual volume.

Table 4-3 Comparative Analysis of Actual Performance to Target and Control Budgets

Memorial Hospital, Anytown, U.S.A.
Patient Business Services Department
Comparative Analysis of Actual Performance to Target and Control Budgets
For the Month Ending September 30, 19x1

	Target Budget	Control Budget	Actual Performance	Variance
Volume (Billings)	6,000	NA	8,000	2,000 Favorable
Volume Adjusted to Actual	NA	8,000	8,000	None
Salary Expense	$6,000	$8,000	$6,000	$2,000 Favorable

compared to the control budget, where volume has been adjusted to actual volume and salary expense adjusted accordingly, using the standard salary rate per billing, there is an unfavorable salary expense variance of $600 (see Table 4-2). Table 4-3 is an example of the impact of the increase of 2,000 billings over the budgeted billing volume of 6,000.

The variable expense budget methodology allows the patient account manager to adjust the budget plan to actual performance volume. Using the methodology, the patient account manager generates a standard rate for each classification of variable expense. That rate is then multiplied by actual volume to develop a control budget. The control budget is then compared to actual performance. This process eliminates variances due to volume differences.

To develop a variable expense budget, each chart of accounts expense item must be classified in one of two categories:[6]

1. fixed expenses: expenses that remain essentially constant in the short run regardless of changes in output volume
2. variable expenses: expenses that tend to vary directly in proportion to changes in output volume.

To illustrate the use of variable expense for budgeting and control, assume that the fixed budget in Table 4-4 is based on a volume of 100,000 billings and 12,000 admissions. Actual billings, however, were 90,000, and actual admissions were 11,250.

The following are the target production standards and rates developed for the admitting and billing clerks and the nonsalary variable expenses:

Position	Production Units	Total FTEs*	Total Hours Paid	Target Production Total Volume	Target Production Volume per Hour (Paid)	Total Expense	Total Expense Rate/Hour Paid (Unit)
Admitting Clerk	number of admissions	3	3,120	12,000	3.8	$18,000	$5.77
Billing Clerk	number of billings	6	6,240	100,000	16.0	$36,000	$5.77
Admitting Supplies	NA	NA	NA	12,000	NA	$12,000	$1.00
Billing Supplies	NA	NA	NA	100,000	NA	$50,000	$ .50

* FTE = Full-time Equivalent
In this illustration: 26 weeks × 40 hrs = 1,040 hrs.

Table 4-5 compares a control budget based on the actual billing volume with actual performance. The key in this approach is to determine in advance which expense classification, fixed or variable, is appropriate.

Table 4–4 Comparative Analysis of Actual Performance to Fixed (Target) Budget

Memorial Hospital, Anytown, U.S.A.
Patient Business Services Department
Comparative Analysis of Actual Performance to Fixed (Target) Budget
For the Six-Month Period Ending June 30, 19x1

	Target Budget	Actual	Variance Fav. (Unfav.)
Volume			
Admissions	12,000	11,250	(750)
Billings	100,000	90,000	(10,000)
Salary Expense			
Management and Supervisor (2)	$ 60,000	$ 59,000	$ 1,000
Executive Secretary (1)	9,000	9,000	None
Billing Clerks (6)	36,000	40,000	(4,000)
Admitting Clerks (3)	18,000	15,000	3,000
Total Salary Expense	$123,000	$123,000	$ None
Nonsalary Expense			
Office Supplies, General	$ 24,000	$ 22,000	$ 2,000
Travel and Meetings	6,000	7,500	(1,500)
Dues and Subscriptions	1,000	1,000	None
Admitting Supplies	12,000	11,500	500
Billing Supplies	50,000	51,000	(1,000)
Depreciation	12,000	12,000	None
Total Nonsalary Expense	$105,000	$105,000	$ None
Total Expense	$228,000	$228,000	$ None

Step 1. Separate the fixed and variable salary expenses in the fixed or target budget as follows:

Fixed Salary Expense		*Variable Salary Expense*	
Management and Supervision	$60,000	Billing Clerks	$36,000
Executive Secretary	9,000	Admitting Clerks	18,000
Total Fixed Salary Expense	$69,000	Total Variable Salary Expense	$54,000

Table 4–5 Comparative Analysis of Actual Performance to Direct Variable Control Budget

Memorial Hospital, Anytown, U.S.A.
Patient Business Services Department
Comparative Analysis of Actual Performance to Direct Variable Control Budget
For the Six-Month Period Ending June 30, 19x1

	Standard Rate	Control Budget	Actual	Variance Fav. (Unfav.)
Volume				
Admissions		11,250	11,250	NA
Billings		90,000	90,000	NA
Fixed Expense				
Salary Expense				
Management and Supervision		$ 60,000	$ 59,000	$ 1,000
Executive Secretary		9,000	9,000	None
Total Fixed Salary Expense		$ 69,000	$ 68,000	$ 1,000
Nonsalary Expense				
Travel and Meetings		$ 6,000	$ 7,500	$ (1,500)
Dues and Subscriptions		1,000	1,000	None
Depreciation		12,000	12,000	None
Total Fixed Nonsalary Expenses		$ 19,000	$ 21,500	$ (2,500)
Total Fixed Expense		$ 88,000	$ 89,500	$ (1,500)
Variable Expense				
Salary Expense				
Billing Clerks	$ .36	$ 32,400	$ 40,000	$ (7,600)
Admitting Clerks	$1.50	16,875	15,000	1,875
Total Variable Salary Expense		$ 49,275	$ 55,000	$ (5,725)
Nonsalary Expense				
Office Supplies, General	$132.60	$ 24,000	$ 22,000	$ 2,000
Admitting Supplies	1.00	11,250	11,500	(250)
Billing Supplies	.50	45,000	51,000	(6,000)
Total Variable Nonsalary Expense		$ 80,250	$ 84,500	$ (4,250)
Total Variable Expense		$129,525	$139,500	$ (9,975)
Total Fixed and Variable Expense		$217,525	$229,000	$(11,475)

Step 2. Establish a standard variable salary rate for each position based on its production units using the following formula:

$$\frac{\text{Total variable salary expense}}{\text{Total relevant production units}} = \text{Standard variable salary rate}$$

Billing Clerks:

$$\frac{\$36,000}{100,000} = \$0.36 \text{ (Standard variable salary rate)}$$

Admitting Clerks:

$$\frac{\$18,000}{12,000} = \$1.50 \text{ (Standard variable salary rate)}$$

Step 3. Separate the fixed and variable nonsalary expenses in the fixed or target budget as follows:

Fixed Nonsalary Expense		*Variable Nonsalary Expense*	
Travel and Meetings	$ 6,000	Office Supplies, General	$24,000
Dues and Subscriptions	1,000	Admitting Supplies	12,000
Depreciation	12,000	Billing Supplies	50,000
Total Fixed Nonsalary Expense	$19,000	Total Variable Nonsalary Expense	$96,000

Step 4. Establish a standard variable nonsalary rate for each distinct nonsalary expense using the following formula:

$$\frac{\text{Total variable nonsalary expense}}{\text{Total relevant production units}} = \text{Standard variable nonsalary rate}$$

Office Supplies, General

Since there is no distinct production unit for general office supplies, the number of calendar days will be used as the production unit in the example:

$$\frac{\$24,000}{181} = \$132.60 \text{ (Standard variable expense rate for general office supplies per calendar day)}$$

Admitting Supplies

$$\frac{\$12,000}{12,000} = \$1.00 \text{ (Standard variable expense rate for admitting supplies per admission)}$$

Billing Supplies

$$\frac{\$50,000}{100,000} = \$0.50 \text{ (Standard variable expense rate for billing supplies per billing)}$$

Step 5. Develop a control budget using the segmented expense classifications and the standard variable expense rates computed in Step 2 and Step 4 adjusted to each relevant production unit as illustrated in Table 4–5, page 78.

VARIANCE ANALYSIS

Once the variances have been identified, the next step is to determine why they occurred. Was the variance due to a change in the hourly rate? Was it due to employee inefficiency or to a production volume variance? These questions can be answered through a process known as variance analysis.

Basically, there are two types of salary variance analysis:

1. efficiency
2. rate

The following process is a step-by-step computation of the salary variances that occurred during one six-month accounting period:

	Admitting Clerks	*Billing Clerks*
I. *Standard or Target*		
1. Standard hourly rate	$5.77	$5.77
2. Standard hours	3,120	6,240
3. Total standard salary expense (line 1 × line 2 = line 3)	$18,000	$36,000

	Admitting Clerks	Billing Clerks
II. Control Standard		
4. Standard hourly rate	$5.77	$5.77
5. Actual hours paid (from Payroll)	2,542	7,272
6. Control standard (line 4 × line 5 = line 6)	$14,667	$41,959
III. Actual Performance		
7. Actual hourly rate	$5.90	$5.50
8. Actual hours paid	2,542	7,272
9. Actual salary expense	$15,000	$40,000
IV. Efficiency Variance		
10. Standard hours	3,120	6,240
11. Actual hours paid	2,542	7,272
12. Hourly variance (line 10 − line 11 = line 12)	578 (favorable)	1,012 (unfavorable)
13. Standard hourly rate	$5.77	$5.77
14. Efficiency variance (line 12 × line 13 = line 14)	$3,335 (favorable)	$5,839 (unfavorable)
V. Rate Variance		
15. Actual hours paid	2,542	7,272
16. Actual hourly rate (from Payroll)	$5.90	$5.50
17. Standard hourly rate	$5.77	$5.77
18. Hourly rate variance (line 16 − line 17 = line 18)	$0.13 (unfavorable)	$0.27 (favorable)
19. Rate variance (line 15 × line 18 = line 19)	$335 (unfavorable)	$1,839 (favorable)

	Admitting Clerks	Billing Clerks
VI. *Total Salary Variances*		
A. Efficiency	$3,335 (favorable)	$5,839 (unfavorable)
B. Rate	$335 (unfavorable)	$1,839 (favorable)
Total Salary Expense Variances	$3,000 (favorable)	$4,000 (unfavorable)

Proof: Compare difference between standard salary expense (line 3) and actual salary expense (line 9):

	Admitting Clerks	Billing Clerks
	$18,000	$36,000
	15,000	40,000
	$3,000	$4,000
	(favorable)	(unfavorable)*
Net variance		$1,000 (unfavorable)

* Adjusted to even numbers.

Nonsalary expenses also have two major types of variance analysis:

1. volume
2. rate

The following procedures comprise a step-by-step approach to computing these variances:

	Admitting Supplies	Billing Supplies
I. *Standard or Target*		
1. Target volume	12,000	100,000
2. Standard expense per unit	$1.00	$0.50
3. Total standard expense (line 1 × line 2 = line 3)	$12,000	$50,000

	Admitting Supplies	Billing Supplies
II. Control Standard		
4. Actual volume	11,250	90,000
5. Standard unit expense	$1.00	$0.50
6. Total control expense (line 4 × line 5 = line 6)	$11,250	$45,000
III. Actual Performance		
7. Actual volume	11,250	90,000
8. Actual unit expense	$1.022	$5.66
9. Actual total expense (line 7 × line 8 = line 9)	$11,500	$51,000
IV. Volume Variance		
10. Target volume	12,000	100,000
11. Actual volume	11,250	90,000
12. Volume variance (line 10 − line 11 = line 12)	750 (favorable)	10,000 (favorable)
13. Standard unit expense	$1.00	$0.50
14. Volume expense variance (line 12 × line 13 = line 14)	$750 (favorable)	$5,000 (favorable)
V. Rate Variance		
15. Standard unit expense	$1.00	$0.50
16. Actual unit expense	$1.022	$5.566
17. Unit expense variance (line 15 − line 16 = line 17)	$0.022 (unfavorable)	$0.066 (unfavorable)
18. Actual volume	11,250	90,000
19. Rate variance (line 17 − line 18 = line 19)	$250 (unfavorable)	$6,000 (unfavorable)

	Admitting Supplies	Billing Supplies
VI. *Total Nonsalary Expense Variances*		
A. Volume	$750 (favorable)	$5,000 (favorable)
B. Rate	$250 (unfavorable)	$6,000 (unfavorable)
Total Nonsalary Expense Variance	$500	$1,000

Proof: Compare difference between standard nonsalary expenses (line 3) and actual nonsalary expenses (line 9):

	$12,000	$50,000
	11,500	51,000
Net variance	$ 500	$1,000
	(favorable)	(unfavorable)

The process outlined above illustrates an application of the variable budgetary control concept, which adjusts the variable expenses in direct proportion to the actual production volume. Some may say, justifiably, that variable salary expenses cannot be adjusted in direct proportion to the volume of work. They would argue that the patient account manager cannot automatically hire a new admitting clerk just because admissions increase by 50 or 100. Conversely, the patient account manager cannot automatically release an admitting clerk when admissions drop by 50 or 100. There is a certain amount of elasticity in any staff during a reasonable period of time. Thus, elasticity tends to create certain plateaus in a patient business services department's staffing requirements. Implementation of a step-variable control creates a "lag factor" which allows the department to adjust to volume variance fluctuations.

The following method may be used to adjust for step-variable components in the situation of admitting and billing clerks in the above case study:

	Admitting Clerks	Billing Clerks
1. Standard or target volume	12,000	100,000
2. Standard or target hours paid	3,120	6,240
3. Standard units per paid hour (line 1 ÷ line 2 = line 3)	3.8	16.0

	Admitting Clerks	Billing Clerks
4. Average hours per week	40	40
5. Weeks per period	26	26
6. Average paid hours per period	1,040	1,040
7. Average production per period (line 3 × line 6 = line 7)	3,952	16,640
8. Standard or target volume	12,000	100,000
9. Actual volume	11,250	90,000
10. Volume variance (line 8 − line 9 = line 10)	750	10,000
11. Average production per period (line 7)	3,952	16,640
12. Average number of steps (to the nearest whole number) (line 11 ÷ line 10 = line 12)	None	One (unfavorable)
13. Average standard hourly rate	$5.77	$5.77
14. Average expense per step (line 6 × line 13 = line 14)	$6,000	$6,000
15. Step-variable adjustment (line 12 × line 14 = line 15)	None	$6,000 (unfavorable)

86 PATIENT ACCOUNT MANAGEMENT

Once the step-variable adjustment has been made, it can be incorporated into the control budget and compared to actual performance as shown in Table 4–6.

Table 4–6 Comparative Analysis of Actual Performance to Step-Variable Control Budget

Memorial Hospital, Anytown, U.S.A.
Patient Business Services Department
Comparative Analysis of Actual Performance to Step-Variable Control Budget
For the 6-Month Period Ending June 30, 19x1

	Control Budget	Actual	Variance FAV (Unpaid)
Volume			
Admissions	11,250	11,250	none
Billings	90,000	90,000	none
Fixed Expense			
Salary Expense	$ 69,000	$ 68,000	$ 1,000
Nonsalary Expense	19,000	21,500	(2,500)
Total Fixed Expense	$ 88,000	$ 89,500	$ (1,500)
Variable Salary Expense			
Standard or Target Salary Expense:			
Admitting Clerks	$ 18,000	$ 15,000	
Billing Clerks	36,000	40,000	
Target Variable Salary Expense	$ 54,000	$ 55,000	
Less: unfavorable step-variable adjustment (line 15)	$ 6,000		
Total Variable Salary Expense	$ 48,000	$ 55,000	$ (7,000)
Variable Nonsalary Expense			
Admitting Supplies	$ 11,250	$ 11,500	$ (250)
Billing Supplies	45,000	51,000	(6,000)
Office Supplies, General	24,000	22,000	2,000
Total Variable Nonsalary Expense	$ 80,250	$ 84,500	$ (4,250)
Total Variable Expense	$128,250	$139,500	$(11,250)
Total Fixed and Variable Expense	$216,250	$229,000	$(12,750)

Table 4–7 is a comparative analysis of the direct variable and step-variable approaches to adjusting variable expenses to match the actual volume of work.

Table 4–7 Comparative Analysis of Actual Performance to Direct Variable and Step-Variable Control Budgets

Memorial Hospital, Anytown, U.S.A.
Patient Business Services Department
Comparative Analysis of Actual Performance to Direct Variable and Step-Variable Control Budgets
For the Six-Month Period Ending June 30, 19x1

	Actual Performance	Direct Variable Control Budget	Step-Variable Control Budget
Volume			
Admissions	11,250	11,250	11,250
Billings	90,000	90,000	90,000
Fixed Expense			
Salary	$ 68,000	$ 69,000	$ 69,000
Nonsalary	20,500	19,000	19,000
Total Fixed Expense	$ 89,500	$ 88,000	$ 88,000
Variable Expense			
Salary	$ 55,000	$ 49,275	$ 48,000
Admitting Supplies	11,500	11,250	11,250
Billing Supplies	51,000	45,000	45,000
Office Supplies, General	22,000	24,000	24,000
Total Variable Expense	$139,500	$129,525	$128,250
Total Fixed and Variable Expense	$228,000	$217,525	$216,250

In summary, developing and using a variable budgetary control system provides the patient account manager with the flexibility to design a system that best fits the needs of his/her own department and institution. Patient account managers and their superiors should work together to classify expenses into the appropriate categories—fixed, direct variable, and step-variable. Once that is done, the patient account manager can work with the financial staff to design management reports that produce the desired results. Variable budgetary control is only one application of expense behavior analysis that can help the patient account manager more effectively manage the patient business services department. Its potential uses are limited only by one's imagination.

NOTES

1. Charles T. Horngren, *Accounting for Management Control: An Introduction* (Englewood Cliffs, N.J.: Prentice-Hall, Inc., 1965), pp. 3–4.
2. Allen G. Herkimer, Jr., *Understanding Hospital Financial Management* (Germantown, Md.: Aspen Systems Corp., 1978), p. 45.
3. L. Vann Seawell, *Hospital Financial Accounting Theory and Practice* (Chicago: Hospital Financial Management Association, 1975), p. 551.
4. Peter F. Drucker, *Management: Tasks, Responsibilities and Practices* (New York: Harper & Row, 1974), p. 120.
5. Herkimer, *Understanding Hospital Financial Management*, p. 60.
6. Ibid., p. 138.

Chapter 5

Developing a Productivity Improvement Program

The goal of every patient account manager should be effective use of available resources such as personnel, supplies, and equipment. Peter Drucker observes that productivity is the first test of management's competence. He defines productivity as "the balance between all factors of production which will give the greatest output for the smallest effort."[1]

For the purposes of this discussion, we will define productivity as "the ration of outputs per unit of inputs over a specific period of time."[2] Outputs will be represented as production units, for example, admissions, accounts billed, discharges, and items handled. Inputs will be represented as employee time, for example, days, hours, and minutes.

An effective productivity improvement program has two major components: (1) work measurement, and (2) performance evaluation. Historically, patient business services departments have been evaluated in terms of whether dollars actually spent exceeded dollars budgeted. If the amount of dollars spent was less than dollars budgeted, management considered the patient account manager's performance to be favorable. On the other hand, the patient account manager's performance was considered to be unfavorable if dollars spent exceeded dollars budgeted. There are two fallacies inherent in this rationale. First, it does not allow for volume variances, and second, it does not take into account the performance of individual employees in the department. (Precise performance evaluation requires that a department's total functions be separated into like tasks for like employees. In addition, the dollar should not be the only measurement used; a unit that reflects changes in work volume is preferable.)

The present system of comparing health care institutions in terms of cost—expressed in dollars—does not permit evaluation of the productivity of the department manager, nor does it stimulate greater productivity. Dollar comparisons yield only an unreliable gross figure which raises more questions than it answers. Worse, only pure rationalization can answer the questions that are raised.[3]

This is not to say that dollar cost comparisons are not necessary; rather, cost comparisons must be supplemented by other quantitative measurements that remain relatively constant over an extended period of time and that reasonably reflect the resources required to produce a specific service or group of services. Production units, or standard units of measurement, are the necessary quantitative measurements. Selection of specific production units will be discussed later in this chapter.

Through effective use of production units, the patient account manager can identify and determine:

- productivity per employee and/or department
- cost per production unit

The use of production units will assist the patient account manager in assigning responsibility for evaluating the effectiveness of the dollars spent to the employees who spent them. Production units also give the manager a means of measuring the department's effectiveness. Although the patient account manager will eventually assign a dollar value to the production unit, the dollar should not be the only measure of the patient business services department's productivity or effectiveness.

Production units are important because they enable the patient account manager to compare actual performance to a planned (budgeted) performance standard. Thus, the first step in developing a productivity improvement program is to identify appropriate production units.

Drucker states that making resources productive is the specific job of management, distinct from other jobs of the manager such as entrepreneurship and administration.[4] The history of management as a distinct social function began 100 years ago with the discovery that resources can be managed for productivity. According to Drucker, only managers—not nature, or laws of economics, or governments—make resources productive. Resources can be made productive in the individual plant, store, hospital, office and so forth. He concludes by saying that individual managers, within their own sphere of responsibility, make resources productive or deprive them of productivity. The patient account manager's sphere of responsibility, of course, is the patient business services department.

PRODUCTION UNIT

As stated earlier, the production unit is a quantitative measurement of work performed. The Department of Health and Human Services' (HHS)

Annual Hospital Report (AHR) relies on a standard unit of measure (SUM) that determines unit cost and revenue to facilitate cost and revenue comparisons among peer group health facilities. According to HHS, the SUM is not to be confused with statistics used to allocate cost of nonrevenue-producing cost centers to each other and to revenue-producing centers.[5] At present, the AHR does not define SUMs nor does it identify a production unit for the patient business services department. However, the California Health Facilities Commission has identified the following units of service:[6]

- patient accounting: $1,000 of gross patient revenue
- credit and collection: $1,000 of gross patient revenue
- admitting: admissions
- data processing: $1,000 of gross patient revenue

In reviewing the information given above, it is important for the patient account manager to remember that a production unit must accurately identify and reflect the service or commodity produced and the amount of resources used to produce the individual unit. For the purposes of this discussion, production units will be divided into two major classes:

1. macro or gross
2. micro or weighted

Macro Production Units

Presently, macro production units are the most commonly used because they require no special studies to determine a weighted value. They are also relatively easy to identify, collect, and audit. Macro production units in the patient business services department include:

- inpatient: admissions
- inpatient: discharges
- outpatient: admissions
- outpatient: discharges

Generally, macro production units do not reflect any amount of resources required to produce a service, nor do they segment a function into separate tasks such as interviewing patients, typing letters, completing admission forms, processing computer bills, or responding to telephone inquiries.

Although macro production units are better than no measurement at all, they do not accurately reflect the amount of work or resources required to perform a given service.

Micro Production Units

Basically, most macro production units can be divided into a number of micro production units. For example, inpatient admissions can be divided into the following micro production units:

- number of preadmission forms completed
- number of patients processed in admitting office *with* preadmission
- number of patients processed in admitting office *without* preadmission
- number of patients interviewed in their rooms
- number of patients escorted or transported to their rooms
- number of contacts with physician's office personnel
- number of physician contacts

The micro production unit reduces the macro production unit to the measurement that most accurately reflects the amount of resources, such as labor, supplies, equipment, and overhead, required to produce the service. Currently, there is no generally accepted micro production unit for the patient business services department. For that matter, there is no clearcut list of functions performed by the department.

SELECTION OF PRODUCTION UNITS

The single most common and workable production unit for evaluating the patient business services department is the amount of average daily revenue uncollected. However, it is not appropriate to use only this index to evaluate the performance of personnel in the department. In fact, there is no single production unit that effectively measures the productivity of personnel in the department. The department has many unique positions with exclusive tasks; consequently, most of the positions have their own production units or sets of units.

The following criteria should be used for selecting any production unit:

- capacity to relate to both fixed and variable behavior of the resources used,
- minimal susceptibility to variables other than volume of work performed,

- ability to be easily understood by employees and management,
- minimal clerical cost, and
- ability to be easily audited and verified for accuracy.

When the patient account manager begins to select production units, he/she may find it necessary to select more than one unit for a given position to account for the fixed and variable components of the functions that are part of that position. For example:

Position: Executive Secretary

Fixed Functions	Production Units
reception duties	number of days worked
secretarial and clerical duties	number of days worked
order and storing of supplies	number of days worked
messenger duties	number of days worked
maintenance of work and reception area	number of days worked
placing and answering of telephone calls	number of days worked

Variable Functions	Production Units
dictation	number of times performed (frequency)
typing and transcription of letters	number of times performed (frequency)
typing, transcription, and distribution of memos	number of times performed (frequency)
filing	number of times performed (frequency)

Other production units might include:

Position	Production Units
Inpatient Admitting Clerk	number of inpatient admissions processed
Outpatient Admitting Clerk	number of outpatients processed
Billing Clerk	number of bills processed by payer

Position
Cashier

Collection Clerk

Production Units
number of cash receipts processed
number of patient account guarantors contacted by (1) mail, and (2) telephone

It is important to establish a standard of acceptable performance for each production unit that is identified. For example:

Production Unit
number of letters typed
number of bills processed
number of cash receipts processed

Performance Standard
no typographical errors
98 percent require no resubmission
maximum of $100 over or short per year

Every job description should list the functions the position includes and acceptable standards of performance for each of those functions (see Exhibit 5–1).

The production unit has four primary uses in the patient business services department:

1. establishing departmental staffing requirements and data for budgetary control
2. monitoring and evaluating departmental and employee performance
3. creating the basis for employee incentive payment plans
4. allocating costs

In selecting the production unit, the patient account manager and the employee must be satisfied that the unit meets all the criteria mentioned above and that it lends itself to forecasting and ease of recording. It is important to stress the need for the employee's involvement in the selection process and his/her acceptance of the unit selected.

STAFFING AND BUDGETARY CONTROL

In establishing staffing requirements, the patient account manager must determine the minimum number of positions that must be filled in order

Exhibit 5-1 Job Description Form

```
┌─────────────────────────────────────────────────────────────────┐
│                  Memorial Hospital, Anytown, U.S.A.             │
│                         Job Description                         │
│                                                                 │
│  Position: _____   Position Number: _____ │
│  Supervisor: _____   Labor Grade: _____ │
│  Department: _____   Exempt: ____  Nonexempt: ___ │
│                                  │                              │
│  Primary Functions               │  Standards of Performance    │
│                                  │                              │
│                                  │                              │
├──────────────────────────────────┼──────────────────────────────┤
│                                  │                              │
│  Secondary Functions             │  Standards of Performance    │
│                                  │                              │
│                                  │                              │
├──────────────────────────────────┴──────────────────────────────┤
│  Approved by: _____   Reviewed with employee:      │
│  Title: _____   Date: _____ 19__ │
│  Date: _____ 19__                               │
│  Employee's signature: _____│
│  Reviewer's signature: _____│
└─────────────────────────────────────────────────────────────────┘
```

to start doing business. These positions, which form the fixed or core component of the department staff, might include:

Fixed or Core Positions	Number Required
Patient Account Manager	1.0
Executive Secretary	1.0
Inpatient Admitting Supervisor	1.0
Outpatient Admitting Supervisor	1.0
Head Cashier	1.0
Billing and Collection Supervisor	<u>1.0</u>
Total Positions	6.0

The number of fixed or core positions should not change when work volume varies until that variance is pronounced or substantial.

96 PATIENT ACCOUNT MANAGEMENT

Most increases in work volume, for example, patient admissions, will be accommodated by the department's variable component. Variable positions might include:

Variable Positions
Billing Clerks
Admitting Clerks
Collection Clerks
Cashiers
File Clerks

The number of variable positions will be determined by the volume of work or production units to be produced. For example, assume that the following production standards have been established:

Variable Positions	*Production Standards*
Billing Clerk	$1,000 accounts billed per month
Admitting Clerk	30 inpatient and outpatient admissions per day
Collection Clerk	500 accounts followed per month
Cashier	50 inpatient and outpatient discharges processed per day
File Clerk	100 inpatient and outpatient discharges processed per day

Further, assume that the hospital has the following volumes of production units during an average month:

number of accounts: 9,000
number of admissions: 3,000
number of inpatient and outpatient discharges: 3,100

The above data would produce the staffing requirement depicted in Table 5-1. To summarize the data presented in the table, the staffing requirement to cope with the hypothetical volume would be:

(1) Positions	(2) Number of Positions	(3) Average Weekly Hours	(4) Number of Hours 2×3=4	(5) Average Hourly Wage	(6) Total Monthly Budget Expense 4×5=6
Fixed	6.0	40	240.0	$33.75	$8,100
Variable	21.3	40	852.0	5.15	4,394
Total	27.3		1,092.0	$11.44	$12,494

Table 5–1 Variable Staffing Requirement

Memorial Hospital, Anytown, U.S.A.
Patient Business Services Department
Variable Staffing Requirement
For Period _____ 19 ___ to _____ 19 ___

(1)	(2)	(3)	(4)	(5)	(6)	(7)	(8)	(9)
Variable Position	Monthly Production Standards	Average Monthly Volume	Required Positions	Average Weekly Hours	Total Number Hours	Average Hourly Wage Excluding Fringe Benefits	Total Monthly Budget Expense	Standard Rate
			3÷2=4		4×5=6		6×7=8	8÷3=9
Billing Clerk	1,000	9,000	9.0	40	360.0	$5.00	$1,800	$.200
Admitting Clerk	900	3,000	3.3	40	132.0	4.80	634	.211
Collection Clerk	1,500	9,000	6.0	40	240.0	5.50	1,320	.147
Cashier	1,500	3,100	2.0	40	80.0	6.00	480	.155
File Clerk	3,000	3,100	1.0	40	40.0	4.00	160	.052
Total Variable Positions, Hours and Expenses			21.3		852.0		$4,394	

Another approach to determining staffing requirements of the patient business services department is the volume-range method illustrated in Figure 5–1. This method establishes relevant ranges of activity, and a fixed number of staff members to serve this range is identified. For example:

Relevant Range of Activity (Number of Accounts)	Number of Billing Clerks Required
0–3,000	5
3,001–5,000	6
5,001–7,000	7
7,001–8,500	8
8,501–9,500	9
9,501–11,000	10
11,001–13,000	11

The two methods described are both ways in which production standards are used to determine staffing levels. The first, the variable approach, uses a standard rate and can be adjusted to actual volume of work. The second, the relevant range of activity (RRA) method, does not provide as precise a measurement; however, it may be the better method because it recognizes that most staffing levels have some elasticity. In other words, a given staff can adapt to a reasonable increase or decrease in work volume for a reasonable amount of time without requiring a change in the number of staff members. Generally, RRA staffing and production levels identify ranges of acceptable performance for minimum and maximum volumes of activity.

In the final analysis, the staffing level methodology selected by the manager depends on what he/she is most comfortable with. The manager may even decide to combine the two methods. No matter which approach is selected, it is important to establish a production standard and staffing rationale; only then can the process of refining performance standards begin.

EVALUATING DEPARTMENTAL PERFORMANCE

Performance evaluation is the process of comparing actual (or historical) performance with budgeted or planned standards to see how closely actual performance matches the planned standard. The information can be expressed in terms of either production or financial statistics.[7]

The performance evaluation process begins with the comparison of budgeted or target volume with the actual volume of work performed (see Table

Productivity Improvement Program 99

Figure 5–1 Volume-Range Staffing Requirement

Memorial Hospital, Anytown, U.S.A.
Patient Business Services Department
Volume-Range Staffing Requirement

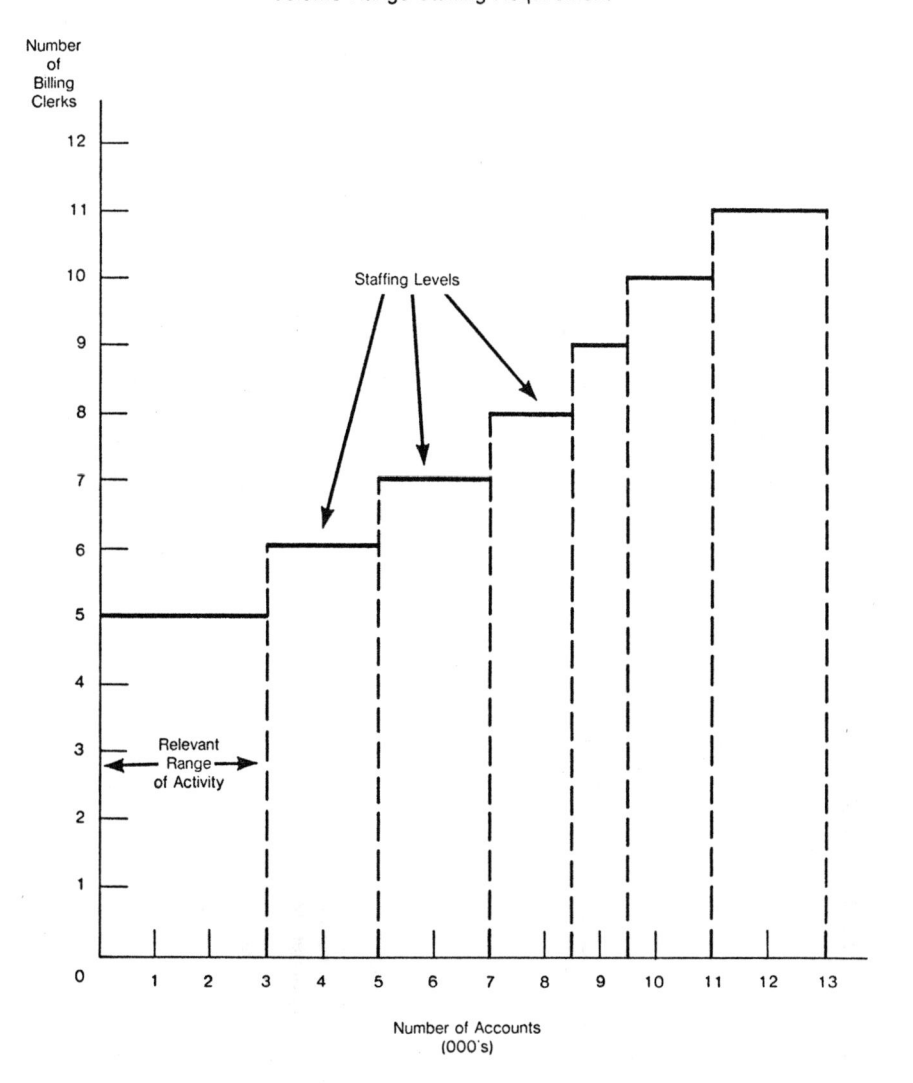

Number of Billing Clerks / Number of Accounts (000's)

Table 5-2 Summary Salary Performance Analysis

Memorial Hospital, Anytown, U.S.A.
Patient Business Services Department
Summary Salary Performance Analysis
For the Month of June 19x1

	Standard Rate	Target Budget	Control Budget	Actual Performance	FAV (UNFAV) Variance $	%
Volume						
Accounts		9,000	8,750	8,750	-0-	-0-
Admissions		3,000	2,875	2,875	-0-	-0-
Discharges		3,100	2,950	2,950	-0-	-0-
Fixed Salaries						
Patient Account Manager		$ 2,500	$ 2,500	$ 2,500	-0-	-0-
Executive Secretary		1,000	1,000	1,100	$(100)	(10.0)
Inpatient Admitting Supervisor		1,200	1,200	1,200	-0-	-0-
Outpatient Admitting Supervisor		1,200	1,200	1,200	100	8.3
Head Cashier		1,000	1,000	1,000	-0-	-0-
Billing/Collection Supervisor		1,200	1,200	1,200	-0-	-0-
Total Fixed Salaries		$ 8,100	$ 8,100	$ 8,100	-0-	-0-
Variable Salaries						
Billing Clerks	$.200	$ 1,800	$ 1,750	$ 1,850	$(100)	(5.7)
Admitting Clerks	.211	634	607	650	(43)	(7.1)
Collection Clerks	.147	1,320	1,286	1,250	36	2.8
Cashier	.155	480	457	480	(23)	(5.0)
File Clerks	.052	160	153	175	(22)	(14.4)
Total Variable Salaries		$ 4,394	$ 4,253	$ 4,405	$ 152	3.6
Total Fixed and Variable Salaries		$12,494	$12,353	$12,505	$ 152	1.2%

5-2). In Table 5-2, the following target and actual volumes for three production units are compared:

	Target	Actual	Variance Number	Variance Percent
Accounts	9,000	8,750	(250)	(2.7)
Admissions	3,000	2,875	(125)	(4.2)
Discharges	3,100	2,950	(150)	(4.8)

An unfavorable volume variance exists for each of the three production units used in the example. To adjust the target budget to compensate for these volume variances, a control budget* must be established that indicates the actual volumes experienced; thus, there are never any volume variances between the control budget and the actual volumes.

The second step is comparison of fixed salary expenses. Because these expenses do not change with volume variances, the target budget expenses can simply be transferred to the control budget. Since most of these employees are paid a fixed salary instead of an hourly wage, variances in this expense category should be minimal.

The third step in performance evaluation is the comparison of the actual variable salary expense with the control budget. The control budget uses a standard rate. The formula for the rate is:

$$\frac{\text{Total variable salary expense}}{\text{Total relevant production units}} = \text{Standard variable salary rate}$$

Graphs are an effective and clear method of communicating performance analysis information. They are also useful for displaying trends, projections, and forecasts. Figures 5-2 and 5-3 are examples of the use of bar graphs to illustrate the differences between the target budget, the control budget, and actual performance in volume and salary expenses based on the information given in Table 5-2.

EMPLOYEE PERFORMANCE EVALUATION

The production unit enables the patient account manager to evaluate an individual employee objectively. Since the production unit is a quantitative

---

* A control budget adjusts the standard rates in a fixed budget to the actual volume of work. As a result, it eliminates variances caused by volume fluctuations.

102 PATIENT ACCOUNT MANAGEMENT

Figure 5–2 Summary Performance Analysis of Volumes

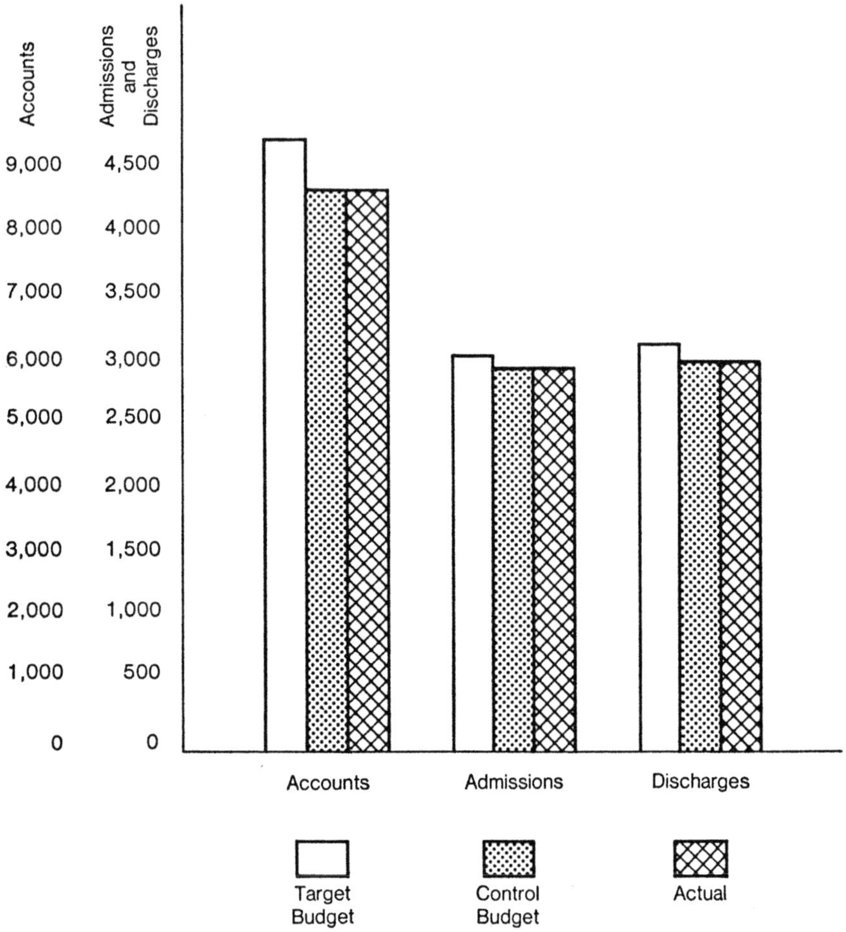

measurement of an employee's production or work, the actual units can be compared readily and objectively to a predetermined employee performance level.

The first step in this application of production units is to work with the employee to be evaluated. Both the employee and the manager must identify the production unit or units that best measure the tasks the employee performs. Once the units have been identified, the manager and subordinate must mutually accept these units as the basis for performance evaluation.

Figure 5–3 Summary Performance Analysis of Salary Expense

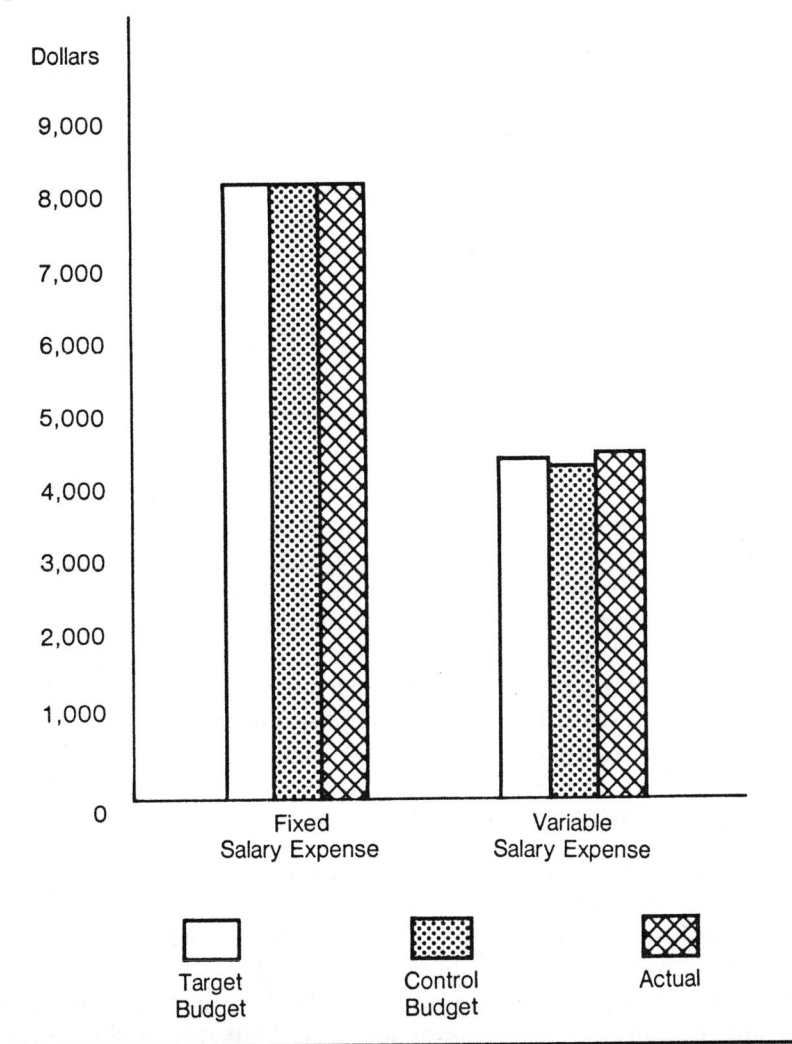

For illustration, assume that the billing clerks have agreed that the production unit used to evaluate their performance should be number of accounts billed. Also assume that the standard of 300 accounts per eight-hour workday has been mutually accepted as a reasonable production standard. (Specific methods used to develop production standards will be discussed later in this chapter.)

104 PATIENT ACCOUNT MANAGEMENT

The predetermined production standard and the actual performance for each billing clerk are then recorded and monitored on a document similar to the one shown in Figure 5–4. In this example, the patient account manager computed the average number of accounts billed per week so that actual performance could be evaluated even before the month was completed. The average weekly actual performances were:

	Accounts Billed		
	1st Week	*2nd Week*	*3rd Week*
Monday	250	350	300
Tuesday	275	325	325
Wednesday	265	275	300
Thursday	285	250	275
Friday	315	275	325
Total	1,390	1,475	1,525
Average	278	295	305

By computing the weekly average actual performance, the patient account manager can readily recognize problem employees and help them improve their performance. The employee performance record should be reviewed, at a minimum, once a month and preferably once a week. Each review period should include discussion of constructive suggestions for productivity improvement. This discussion should not be limited to the manager giving suggestions; rather, these sessions should be two-way exchanges of ideas on how to improve productivity.

EMPLOYEE INCENTIVE PLANS

Third party reimbursement systems have indirectly penalized hospitals and their managers for being efficient and keeping costs down. As a result, there has been little motivation or incentive to operate efficiently. Some lack of motivation still exists, but it is becoming increasingly obvious that only efficient hospitals can survive. Hospitals whose managers can improve productivity, motivate employees, and reward efficiency will be the ones that continue to operate. For this reason, it is imperative that the patient account manager seriously consider implementing an employee incentive plan to reward the efficient employee and motivate the less efficient employee.

A number of employee incentive plans are already in use in the hospital industry. Some reward only the department manager; some reward the entire department staff; and others reward individual high performers. In fact, the cornerstone of employee incentive plans should be some method of rewarding the high performer.

Figure 5-4 Employee Performance Record

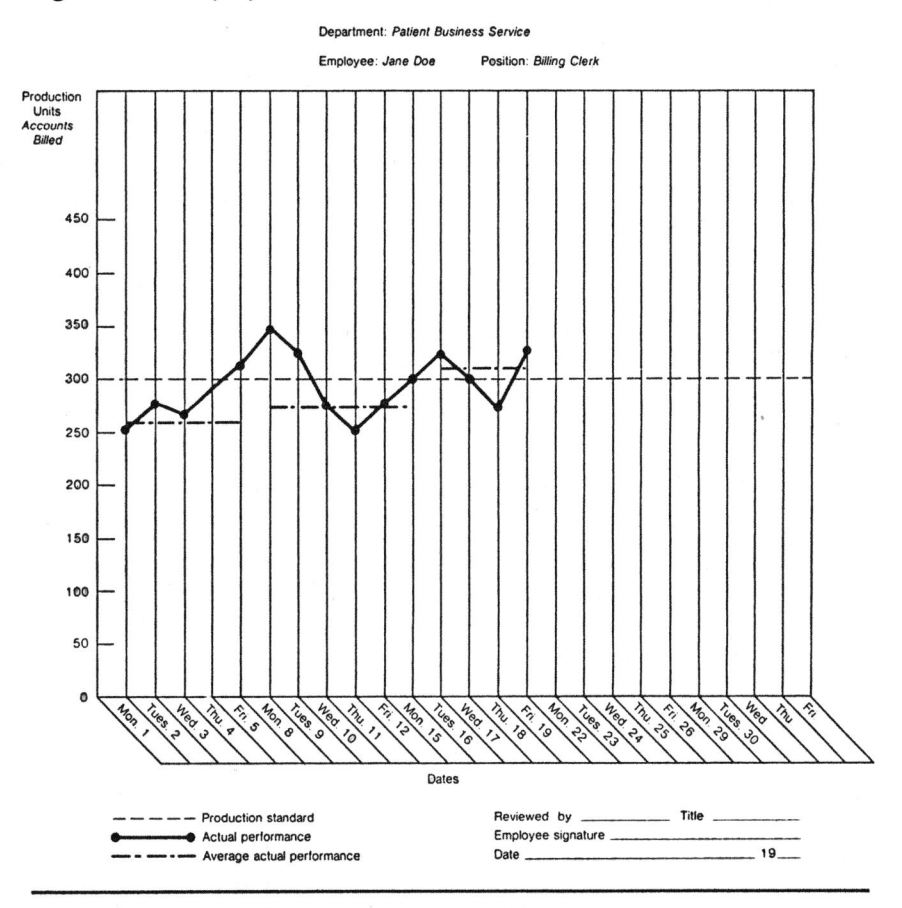

Department: *Patient Business Service*
Employee: *Jane Doe*   Position: *Billing Clerk*

[Chart: Production Units / Accounts Billed plotted against dates Mon 1 through Fri, with y-axis from 0 to 450. Legend indicates: Production standard (dashed), Actual performance (solid with dots), Average actual performance (dash-dot). Fields below: Reviewed by ___ Title ___, Employee signature ___, Date ___ 19__]

The following terms are essential to understanding employee incentive plans:

> Target Level:[8]   The standard of personnel performance that reflects the work pace of a motivated worker with sufficient skill and capability, performing a specified task under capable supervision. This production level takes into account normal fatigue and delay time and represents a pace that can be maintained without a harmful effect on the worker or his/her work.

Reward Level:[9] The standard performance that reflects the work pace established by management as being desirable. The reward level might be set ten percent higher than the target level and is the level at which incentive rewards begin.

Both target levels and reward levels are usually expressed in terms of production units per person per workday. For example:

- admitting: weighted admissions per person hour
- credit: weighted admissions per person hour
- cashier: weighted discharges and receipts per workday
- billing: accounts billed per workday

To illustrate the use of the production unit in an employee incentive plan, assume that the following production levels were established for the billing clerks:

- target level: 285 accounts billed per workday
- reward level: 300 accounts billed per workday

Using the actual average performance data given on page 104, the patient account manager can compute employee compensation in the following manner:

(1) Week	(2) Actual Performances	(3) Target Level	(4) Performance Factor (2÷3=4)	(5) Regular Hourly Wage	(6) Incentive Hourly Wage (4×5=6)
1st	278	285	97.5%	$5.00	$4.875
2nd	295	285	103.5%	$5.00	$5.175
3rd	305	285	107.0%	$5.00	$5.350

Employee incentive plans can be designed in numerous ways. However, no matter how sophisticated they are, employee incentive plans cannot substitute for effective management. Groner states that incentives will make good supervisors better, but they are not a crutch that can make up for the lack of sound supervisory systems. Further, weak supervisors generally will be ineffective in using incentive plans as motivators.[10]

COST ALLOCATION

A dictionary defines allocation as a means of distributing, assigning, or sharing.[11] A production unit or statistic is used to distribute or allocate costs in the hospital's cost finding process. Cost finding, which will be discussed in Chapter 8, has been defined as the apportionment or allocation of the costs of the nonrevenue-producing cost centers to each other and to the revenue-producing centers on the basis of statistical data that measure the amount of service rendered by each center to other centers.[12] The accuracy of cost finding results depends to a great degree on the selection of the production unit and the order of distribution. Although no general consensus exists as to which production unit is most appropriate, the following examples are recommended:

California Hospital Association:[13]
patient accounting: $1,000 of gross patient revenue
credit and collection: $1,000 of gross patient revenue
admitting: admissions

Connecticut Hospital Association:[14]
patient billing and collection: gross revenue by department
admitting: discharges by service

American Hospital Association:[15]
patient accounting: number of patient days
admitting: number of admissions

As shown, there is no one definite production unit on which to base cost allocation. Each hospital should strive for the degree of sophistication it can economically justify in view of its goals and objectives.

The patient account manager is responsible for selecting and/or recommending production units that most equitably measure services rendered by the patient business services department and in turn maximize the hospital's reimbursement for those services. Since cost allocation is an integral part of the rate setting process, it is imperative that the production units be thoroughly tested to ensure that they accurately represent the department's total costs. Equally important is that the production unit selected for cost allocation does not have to be the same as the production unit used to evaluate employee performance. Indeed, in all probability they will not be the same.

DEVELOPMENT OF PRODUCTION STANDARDS

There are numerous systems used to develop production standards. These systems fall into two major groups:

1. predetermined
2. involvement

The predetermined production standard approach uses motion time measurement (MTM) studies that require trained industrial or management engineering personnel to perform detailed studies. Since this approach is highly detailed, it is very sensitive to any change in work procedure and must be adjusted accordingly. This approach does have the advantage of being a proven scientific method. However, at times, this highly impersonal, scientific approach can be extremely costly and relatively difficult to implement. Many employees feel that the production standards that result from this method are not relevant to their work since they were not involved in establishing the standards.

The involvement approach to developing production standards requires the direct involvement of the employees who will be evaluated. Historical information, self-logging, and time studies of relevant functions are some of the techniques used in the involvement approach to setting production standards.

Experiments and experience indicate that production standards established through employee involvement are more readily accepted by employees because:[16]

- the standards are derived from actual department performance
- the department manager and department personnel actually participate in the development of the standards
- the time standards and the system as a whole are relatively simple and easy to understand

How To Develop Production Standards

The following step-by-step procedure can be used to develop production standards:

Step I. Develop the normal task time per production unit for each employee position. The normal time is the average time a qualified employee takes under normal circumstances to perform a task or group of tasks; no provision is made for personal, fatigue, and delay (PFD) time.

1. Classify all tasks into productive work for each production unit and respective PFD factor. This is completed before the self-logging process begins (see Table 5-3).

2. Calculate the normal time for each task by purging the nonrepresentative logged time from the raw data (see the Daily Employee Self-Logging Worksheet shown in Exhibit 5-2) and computing the average of all the logged task times (see Tables 5-4 and 5-5). The average, which is calculated by dividing the total of all the individual task times by the number of occurrences, represents the normal time it should take an average experienced employee to perform the task. It should not require any adjustment unless there is a change in the department methods, procedures, or equipment.

3. Develop task frequency mix factors to indicate the number of times a task is performed per production unit by paid employees on a normal shift (see Tables 5-4 and 5-5). (A task that constitutes part of a production unit need not be performed every time the unit occurs.) This percentage figure reflects the number of times it is performed.

4. Multiply normal task times by frequency/mix factors to compute the average normal task time per production unit. For example, if an admitting

Table 5-3 Departmental Task List

Memorial Hospital, Anytown, U.S.A.
Departmental Task List

Department: *Admitting*   Section: *Inpatient Admitting*

TASK

No.	Description	Production Unit
10	file admissions, pull preadmissions, and maintain files	patient admitted
11	log inpatient admission	patient admitted
12	type and distribute reports	patient admitted
13	order and store supplies	week
15	secretarial, clerical duties	week
16	receptionist duties	week
17	messenger duties	week
20	clean up area, assist others	week
21	answer telephone, telephone reports	week

Exhibit 5-2 Daily Employee Self-Logging Worksheet

Memorial Hospital, Anytown, U.S.A.
Daily Employee Self-Logging Worksheet

Employee Name _____
Position _____
Department _____
Section _____
Date _____ 19 __

Task No.	Task Description & Equipment	Units	Time Start	Time Stop	Minutes	Task No.	Task Description & Equipment	Units	Time Start	Time Stop	Minutes
SUBTOTAL						SUBTOTAL					
						TOTAL					

Table 5–4 Standard Time Development Worksheet

Memorial Hospital, Anytown, U.S.A.
Standard Time Development Worksheet

Department: *Admitting* Section: *Inpatient Admitting*
Production Unit: *Patients Admitted* Employee Position: *Admitting Clerk*
Date: _____ 19__

\ TASK \		Normal Minutes Per Task	Frequency Per Production Unit	Refer To Matrix	Normal Minutes Per Production Unit
No.	Description				
11	log inpatient admissions	.528	1.00	2A	.528
12	type and distribute reports	3.451	1.00	3A	3.451
10	file admissions, pull preadmissions, and maintain files	4.579	1.00	4A	4.579
Total Normal Minutes per Production Unit					8.558
Standard Hours per Production Unit (including 6.4% PFD factor)					.152

---

clerk admits 50 percent of all patients admitted on a normal shift and the normal task time is ten minutes, the normal task time average per production unit, that is, number of admissions, is 50 percent of ten minutes or five minutes.

Step II. Using the standard time development sheets (Tables 5–4, page 111; and 5–5, page 112), calculate standard production unit time for each employee classification. Standard production unit time is the total of all normal task time per production unit plus an allowance for personal, fatigue, and delay (PFD) time. To calculate standard production unit time, follow these steps:

1. Total the normal task times for all the tasks that make up the production unit.

2. Develop a PFD factor to convert normal time to standard time. The PFD factor calculation is based on actual time recorded during a self-logging period, supervisor's estimates, and hospital policy guidelines. The formula is:

$$\text{PFD factor \%} = \frac{\text{Personal time}}{\text{Reported productive time} + \text{delay time}}$$

112 PATIENT ACCOUNT MANAGEMENT

Table 5–5 Standard Time Development Worksheet

Memorial Hospital, Anytown, U.S.A.
Standard Time Development Worksheet

Department: *Admitting* Section: *Inpatient Admitting*
Production Unit: *Week* Employee Position: *Admitting Clerk*
Date: _____ 19__

TASK No.	Description	Normal Minutes Per Task	Frequency Per Production Unit	Refer To Matrix	Normal Minutes Per Production Unit
13 15 16	order and store supplies secretarial, clerical duties receptionist duties	5.323	1.00		5.323
17	messenger duties	572	1.00		572
20	clean up area, assist others	288	1.00		288
21	answer telephone, telephone reports	761	1.00		761
Total Normal Minutes per Production Unit					6.944
Standard Hours per Production Unit (including 6.4% PFD factor)					123.1

3. To compute the standard production unit time, multiply the total normal task time by the PFD factor as follows:

$$\text{Standard production unit time} = \text{Normal production time} \times \text{PFD factor}$$

Step III. Since standard minutes may be too cumbersome for developing staffing requirements, convert the standard minutes to standard hours as follows:

$$\frac{\text{Standard}}{\text{production unit hour}} = \frac{\text{Total standard production unit minutes}}{60}$$

Step IV. Since an employee cannot always perform his/her tasks in the normal time, nor be engaged in productive tasks 100 percent of the working day, a performance factor is calculated to make allowances for:

- unavoidable delays, such as waiting for a patient, doctor, etc.
- normal fluctuations in the workflow
- abnormal occurrences encountered during the performance of productive work

The formula for calculating the performance factor is:

$$\text{Performance factor \%} = \frac{\text{Normal productive time}}{\text{Total reported productive time} + \text{delay time}}$$

Step V. Next, compute the adjusted standard hours required (ASHR). The ASHR represents the total paid work hours that a department or section should require to perform a given volume of work over a specified period of time during the regularly scheduled shift (excluding on-call and non-normal hours worked). (See Table 5–6.) The formula to compute the ASHR is:

$$\text{ASHR} = \frac{\text{Total standard hours required}}{\text{Performance factor}}$$

Step VI. The sixth step is to identify and total all unmeasurable time, such as on-call hours, and all other time that must be spent or used even if the workload is negligible.

Step VII. The final calculation determines the target production level (TPL) for each employee classification in each department or section. The target production level is the result of the calculations of Steps V and VI. The formula is:

$$\begin{array}{c}\text{Adjusted standard}\\\text{hours produced}\end{array} + \begin{array}{c}\text{Other scheduled}\\\text{staff hours}\end{array} + \begin{array}{c}\text{On-call scheduled}\\\text{hours}\end{array}$$

$$= \text{TPL for all reporting units}$$

The self-logging, employee involvement method is not designed to be a management tool to be used for external evaluation and comparison of performance. Rather, it is an internal management tool that enables the

Table 5–6 Performance Factor Calculation Worksheet

Memorial Hospital, Anytown, U.S.A.
Performance Factor Calculation Worksheet

Department: *Admitting*   Section: *Inpatient Admitting*
                           Date: _____ 19__

Number of Personnel Measured: Full Time _____
                                Part Time _____
                      Unmeasured: Administrative _____
                                  Physician _____

		Hours
1. Total paid hours for all measured personnel		16,622
2. Less hours paid for but not measured Vacation Holiday Illness, Absence Others* On-Call—Not Worked On-Call—Worked	Total #2	1,511
3. Total hours applied to measured work (#1 less #2)		15,111

4. Standard hours produced—all employee classifications:

Reporting Unit (Specify)	Standard Hours Per Reporting Units (A)	Number of Reporting Units (B)	Standard Hours Produced (A × B)
Inpatient Admissions	.152	46.800	7,113
Weeks	123.1	52	6,401

Total hours Produced #4	13,514
Variance hours (#3 less #4)	1,597
5. Performance factor $\dfrac{\text{(Total \#4)}}{\text{(Total \#3)}}$	89.4

*Example: Special assignment hours such as attending conference outside hospital by "measured" employee.

patient account manager to measure and evaluate employee and departmental performance. Again, graphs are an excellent medium for depicting production standards and performance. The production trend chart shown in Figure 5-5 shows how a graph can be used to convey this information.

In summary, the scientific exactness of a production standard is not as important as its acceptance and use by both supervisor and subordinate. The key point is that even loosely defined production standards that are accepted, used, and refined are preferable to rejected, albeit scientifically accurate, standards or nonexistent standards. Production standards are

Figure 5-5 Production Trend Chart

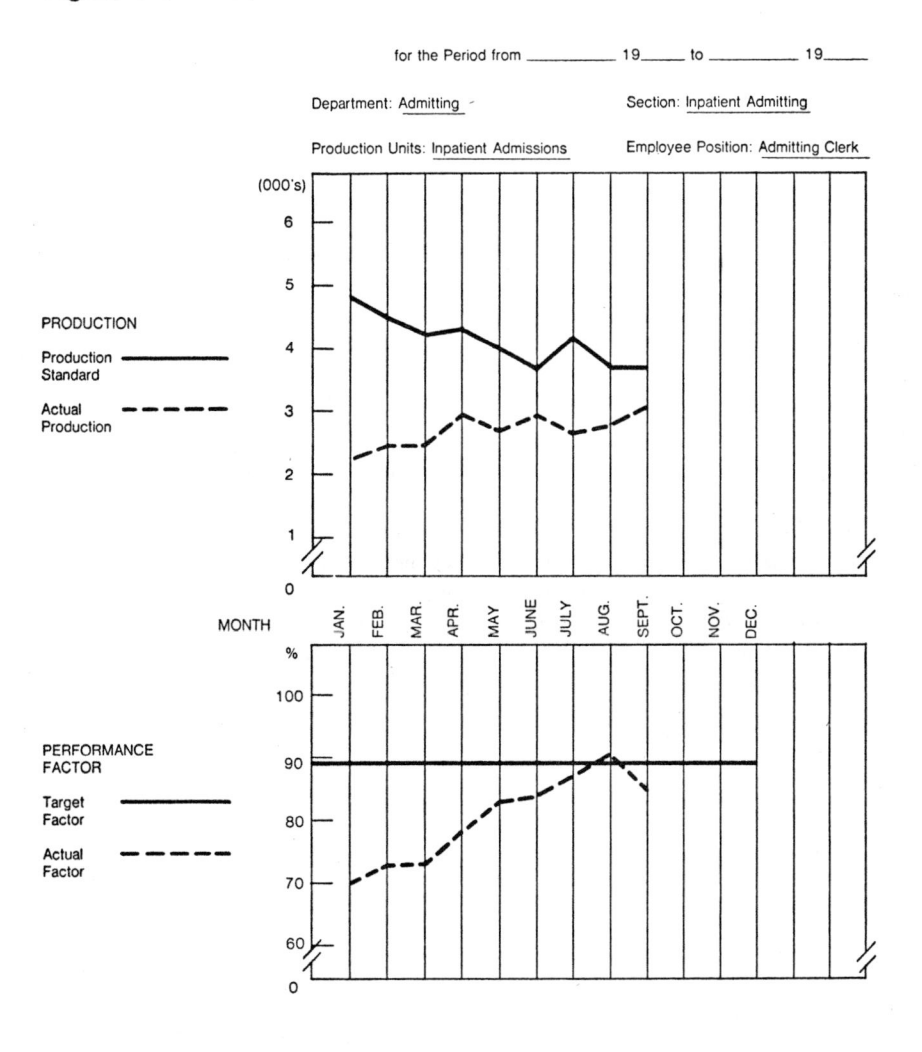

merely a means of measuring actual performance against what the patient account manager desires and expects from a given work effort or dollar expenditure. Productivity is the first test of management's competence and, it should be added, labor's competence as well.

NOTES

1. Peter F. Drucker, *Management Tasks, Responsibilities, Practices* (New York: Harper & Row, 1974), p. 68.
2. Allen G. Herkimer, Jr., *Understanding Hospital Financial Management* (Germantown, Md.: Aspen Systems Corp., 1978), p. 77.
3. Allen G. Herkimer, Jr., *Concepts in Hospital Financial Management*, 2nd ed. (Northridge, Calif.: Alfa Associates, Inc., 1973), p. 55.
4. Peter F. Drucker, *Managing in Turbulent Times* (New York: Harper & Row, 1980), p. 14.
5. *Annual Hospital Report*, February 20, 1980 draft (Washington D.C.: United States Department of Health and Human Services, Health Care Financing Administration), p. 3.26.
6. *Budgeting Manual* (Sacramento, Calif.: California Health Facilities Commission, 1977), p. 39.
7. Herkimer, *Understanding Hospital Financial Management*, p. 82.
8. Patrick N. Groner, *Cost Containment through Employee Incentive Programs* (Germantown, Md.: Aspen Systems Corp., 1977), p. 52.
9. Ibid., p. 52.
10. Ibid., p. 98.
11. *Thorndike-Barnhart Comprehensive Desk Dictionary* (Garden City, N.Y.: Doubleday & Co., 1967), p. 54.
12. *Cost Finding and Rate Setting for Hospitals* (Chicago: American Hospital Association, 1968), p. 1.
13. California Health Facilities Commission, *Budgeting Manual*, p. 39.
14. *Accounting Manual* (New Haven, Conn.: Connecticut Hospital Association, 1974), p. 15.
15. *Cost Finding and Rate Setting for Hospitals*, p. 35.
16. Allen G. Herkimer, Jr., "Developing Production Standards for Physician-Directed Hospital Department," Master's Thesis, University of Bridgeport, 1972.

Chapter 6
The Budgetary Control System

The budgetary control system has been defined as a process that guides and assists all levels of hospital management in achieving established financial and statistical objectives, goals, and performance standards. An effectively installed budgetary control system helps to assure management that it is on its planned course of action and that it is realizing planned results from operations.[1] The budget has been described as a plan of authorized costs a department will expend in performing its function during the next year.[2]

To obtain the correct perspective on the budgetary control system, it is necessary to examine several key words and phrases:

- process
- assist
- achieve
- financial and statistical
- performance standards
- planned course
- results
- authorized
- next year

The word "process" implies that budgetary control is an ongoing, day-to-day series of functions and tasks that must be continually performed, evaluated, and monitored in order to identify weaknesses and strengths within the system. The budgetary control system is a management tool that has evolved into a management style that makes all levels of management acutely aware of their respective goals, objectives, and desired results.

The budgetary control system is designed to assist management in obtaining planned results; it cannot obtain these results without the involvement of people. An internationally known industrialist, George Ball, once observed that nations prosper when their economic systems unleash the full measure of their people's energy, ability, character, and initiative, and allow them the freedom to make the most of their opportunities.[3] In hospitals, as in nations, people must be given a reasonable degree of freedom to assist management and to become involved in order for results to be obtained.

Achievement is the hallmark of successful planning. The patient account manager will never know what has been achieved unless specific goals and objectives are identified. These goals and objectives must be spelled out and quantified in order to evaluate the period's performance in terms of achieving desired results.

Although the budgetary control system is not exclusively financial—it has many other components such as goals and objectives—the quantitative statistics, such as patient days and patient admissions, never change. The net result of the budgetary control system is a documented financial plan based on sound logic and a firm, quantifiable statistical base.

Performance or production standards are the criteria that management establishes before a specific task is actually performed. These standards are another way to describe management's desired results, and they form the basis on which management evaluates actual performance. To organize and staff effectively, the patient account manager must start with proper delegation and then establish the quality level at which individuals are expected to perform. These expected levels of performance or production standards have been discussed in detail in Chapter 5.

The budgetary control system charts a planned course of action with expressed desired results. Top management justifiably expects a planned course of action and a set of planned results. The patient account manager should plot this course of action for the patient business services department. To plan effectively, the patient account manager must seek input from the supervisors (multilateral) who report to him or her and indirectly from their subordinates. It is foolhardy for the patient account manager to plan the department's course of action (unilateral) and to identify desired results without full consultation with, and agreement of, his or her supervisory staff. The budgetary control system requires teamwork.

Management for results begins with the analysis of result areas—in other words, definition of the department's output or services generated. For example, in the patient business services department, output units might include:

- patients admitted
- bills processed
- interviews conducted

Drucker tells us that concentration is the key to economic results.[4] He states that economic results require managers to concentrate their efforts on the smallest number of products or services that will produce the largest amount of revenue. He also observes that managers must minimize the amount of attention devoted to services that are not cost effective because their volume is too small or too splintered. The word "concentration" is key in the management for results concept. Before the concentration process can begin, however, one must identify desired results. This step is a prerequisite for the entire budgetary control system.

In most hospitals, an approved budget is an authorized financial plan and course of action that the hospital's board of trustees (directors) and chief executive officer refer to department managers, including the patient account manager, for implementation. Ideally, the patient account manager has been actively involved in identifying the department's objectives, goals, volume, and financial and performance standards for incorporation in the budget.

The last key phrase in understanding the budgetary control system is "next year." Predicting the future entails a considerable amount of risk for the forecaster—in this case, the patient account manager. This is especially true when the hospital depends on the forecast to know what its cash inflow will be for the next 12 months, the next 3 years, and so forth.. The patient account manager's role in this process is critical for two reasons. First, his/her forecast has a short-run impact on the financial plan of the patient business services department. Second, and more important, is its impact on the more sensitive task of projecting the hospital's total cash inflow. Obviously, any major miscalculation will adversely affect the entire hospital and its service area and patients. In fact, the ultimate survival of the hospital may depend on accurate cash flow forecasting.

To summarize, the budgetary control system is a management process that uses the optimum skills of the hospital's total management team in a well-documented, forward-thinking plan designed to carry out the hospital's mission and to achieve its goals and objectives. An essential part of the hospitalwide strategic plan is the synchronization of each department's individual plan with the overall plan.

Critical to the successful implementation and operation of the budgetary control system is the element of "humantology."[5] Experience in observing many well-managed departments and hospitals leads to the conclusion that the organized efforts of a group of individuals, rather than individual genius, achieve effective operations. Through organization, tasks are divided so that the work can be done properly, performance supervised, and results controlled.[6]

ROLE OF THE PATIENT ACCOUNT MANAGER

Each department manager must be actively involved in the development of his/her department's financial plan—the budget. The patient account manager should also play a leading role in cash forecasting and management for the entire hospital, a responsibility that is discussed more fully in Chapter 10.

The patient account manager's position is clearly the most critical in the process of setting objectives and goals for the patient business services department because it links the plans of the hospital's board and administration with the work of the department staff. If the patient account manager fails to understand the plan, it will never filter down to the individual employee correctly. Perhaps the worst situation would occur when the patient account manager understands the plan but fails to communicate appropriate information to his/her staff. Effective two-way communication is essential. Without complete and active cooperation, as well as total commitment to the plan on the part of the patient account manager and his/her staff, the budgetary control system cannot succeed. There must be no credibility gap between management and employees.

Recently, patient account managers have come to recognize their roles as leaders of people, not just skilled technicians. In this leadership role, the manager should be able to distinguish between the goal-oriented employee and the task-oriented employee. The goal-oriented employee does not like close supervision while working but is interested in finding out results. The goal-oriented employee is eager to accept challenges, wants definite goals, and feels a need to reach objectives. The task-oriented employee, on the other hand, just wants to do his/her particular job and has little interest in overall results. By recognizing these differences, the patient account manager is better equipped to set realistic goals for individual employees and for the department.

FUNCTIONAL AND RESPONSIBILITY BUDGETING

Broadly speaking, there are two major approaches to the budgetary control system. One approach, the functional accounting and budgeting approach, assigns costs and revenues to a specific function, such as admitting, billing, and collection, without regard to who is responsible for the management of the function. Theoretically, the primary purpose of functional accounting and budgeting is to enable the analyst to compare the functional costs of one hospital with the same functional costs in another institution. In theory, the approach seems reasonable; in practice, the approach has proven to be relatively difficult to apply.

The second approach, responsibility accounting and budgeting, is the most universally accepted method because its primary purpose is to control costs and revenues. This system allocates costs and revenues in line with the organization's structure and delegation of responsibility and authority. It is based on the premise that each manager should be held accountable for a specific responsibility center and its related controllable costs and revenues.

To illustrate how these two budgeting systems work, assume that the following inpatient and outpatient functions have been identified for the patient business services department (see Figure 6–1):

- preadmission
- admitting

Figure 6–1 Functions of the Patient Business Services Department, Memorial Hospital, Anytown, U.S.A.

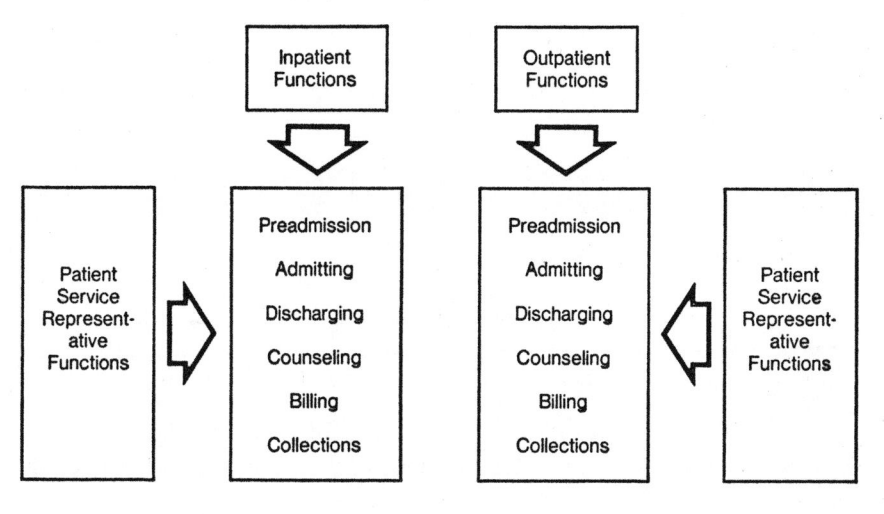

122 PATIENT ACCOUNT MANAGEMENT

- discharging
- counseling
- billing
- collections

Further assume that a patient service representative (PSR) system organizational structure (see Figure 6–2) has replaced the traditional patient business services department structure (see Figure 6–3). In this system, one PSR unit performs all the functions previously handled by separate units such as billing, admitting, and so forth. If a functional accounting and budgeting system were used, time and related expenses would have to be reallocated from the PSR responsibility center to an individual functional area. On the other hand, under the responsibility accounting and budgeting system, each PSR unit would be designated a responsibility center regardless of the organizational structure, and one individual would be held accountable for costs and revenues generated by that center. It should be emphasized that it is totally unacceptable in the budgetary control system for a department manager or supervisor to be held accountable for costs incurred or caused by another individual or department.

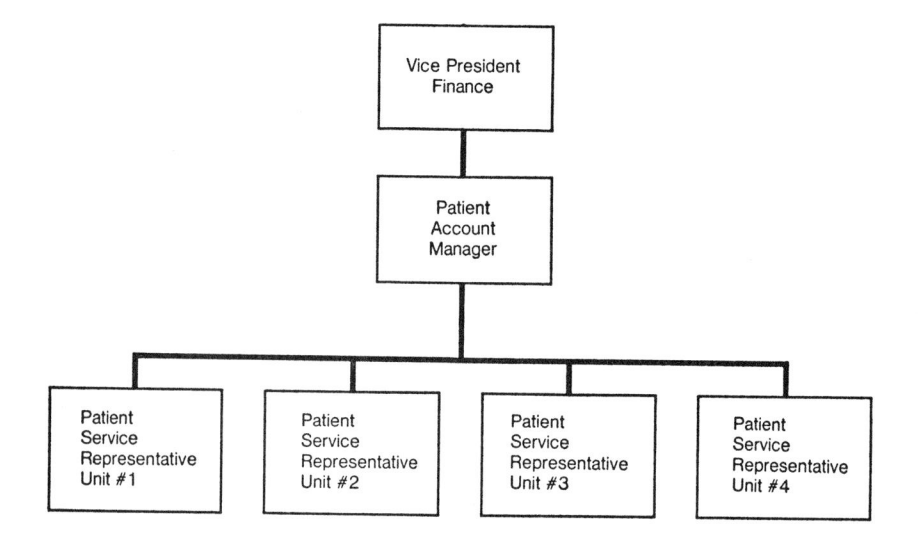

Figure 6–2 PSR—Patient Business Services Department Organizational Structure, Memorial Hospital, Anytown, U.S.A.

```
                    Vice President
                       Finance
                          |
                      Patient
                      Account
                      Manager
                          |
    ┌─────────────┬───────┴───────┬─────────────┐
  Patient       Patient         Patient       Patient
  Service       Service         Service       Service
Representative Representative Representative Representative
  Unit #1       Unit #2         Unit #3       Unit #4
```

Figure 6–3 Traditional Patient Business Services Department Organizational Structure, Memorial Hospital, Anytown, U.S.A.

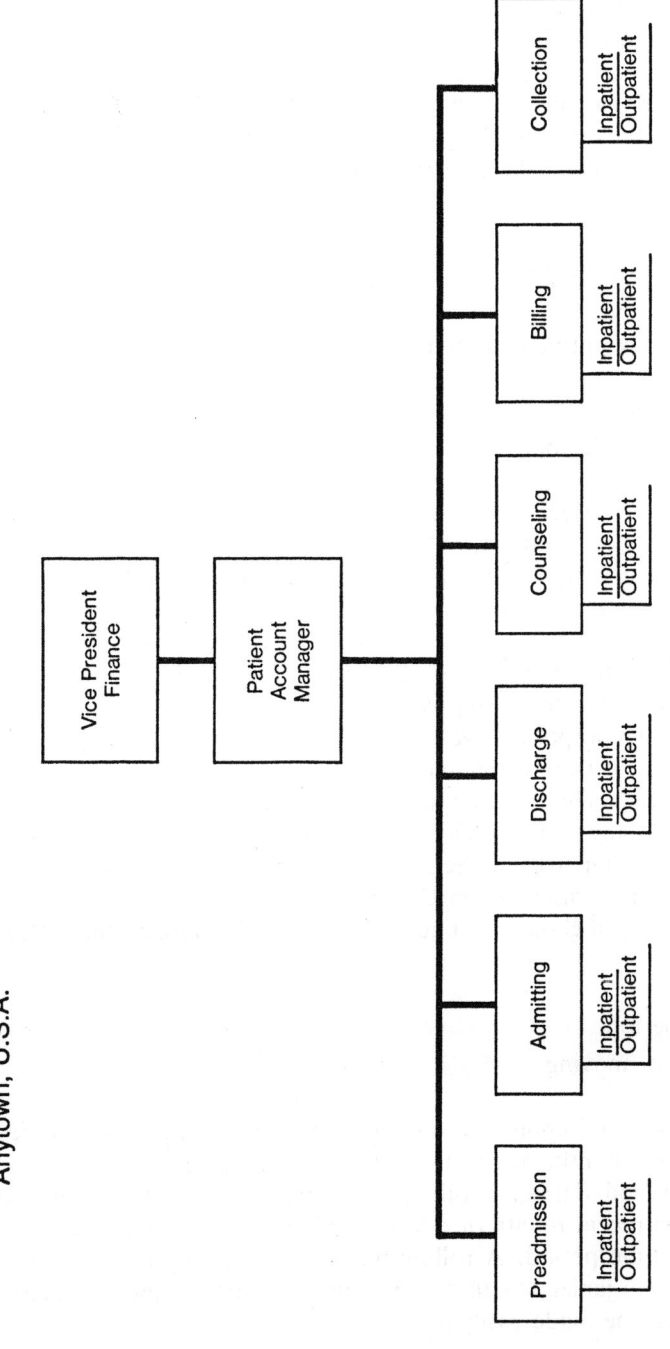

124 PATIENT ACCOUNT MANAGEMENT

If management's primary purpose is to control costs and to operate effectively, responsibility accounting and budgeting is the approach to use. On the other hand, if management is more concerned with comparing its costs with another institution's costs, perhaps functional accounting and budgeting is the appropriate system. Throughout this book, references to budgeting and budgetary control systems refer only to responsibility accounting and budgeting.

TYPES OF BUDGETS

There are two primary systems of budgeting in the hospital setting:

- fixed or target
- variable or flexible

The fixed or target budget system does not distinguish between cost behaviors, that is, fixed, variable, or step-variable, of a department's cost items (see Chapter 4). Rather, all costs are considered fixed for the budget's projected volume of activity.

The variable or flexible system of budgeting, on the other hand, requires each cost item to be identified as one of the following three types: (1) fixed; (2) variable; or (3) step-variable.

The primary purpose of variable budgeting is to allow the analyst or manager to adjust the variable expense items according to the actual volume of activity. The fixed approach does not allow for this adjustment; consequently, any budget variance resulting from volume changes must be rationalized rather than mathematically adjusted. The application of variable budgeting is discussed in Chapter 7.

Another way of classifying budgeting systems is based on time. Budgets may be:

- fixed period
- rolling or moving

The fixed period approach to budgeting identifies a period of time, for example, one month, one year, or two years, and develops a budget to cover that period of time. A rolling or moving budget deletes the projection for the most recent month or quarter and extends the budget by the corresponding time period. A rolling budget is especially effective in a department or organization that experiences dynamic growth because adjustments can be made easily and routinely.

Other types of budgets include:

- appropriations budget
- program or project budget
- zero-base budget

The appropriations budget is used primarily by government agencies and municipalities. In this approach, fixed expenditures are established for each department or cost center. Expense overruns or underruns cannot be transferred to another department without formal approval. This approach to budgeting is relatively archaic due to its cumbersome methodology and lack of incentive to control costs.

The program budget, also called a project budget, is designed to project costs and revenues for one specific program, for example, inhouse collection of accounts. This approach to budgeting is especially effective when management wants to monitor the costs and revenues of a new program or project. The program budget is usually developed apart from the traditional budgetary control system and is simply a supplement to the overall budget. The program budget approach is a very effective management tool for determining the cost/benefit of a specific new program or project, but it should never be considered a replacement for the responsibility budgetary control system.[7]

Zero-base budgeting adopts the premise that a department or program will continue only as long as it can justify its existence. The approach has two basic steps:

1. development of decision packages
2. ranking of decision packages

Once decision packages are developed and ranked in order of priority, management can allocate resources accordingly—funding the most important decision packages whether they are new or existing. The final budget is developed by sorting decision packages approved for funding into appropriate budget units and totaling the cost of individual packages to produce the budget for each unit or department.[8]

In summary, the Budgeting Classification Tree (Figure 6–4) illustrates the various types and approaches which can be used in the budgetary control process.

THE BUDGETARY CONTROL SYSTEM

As long as hospitals and other organizations exist, there will be variations in the approaches and techniques of budgetary control. However, there

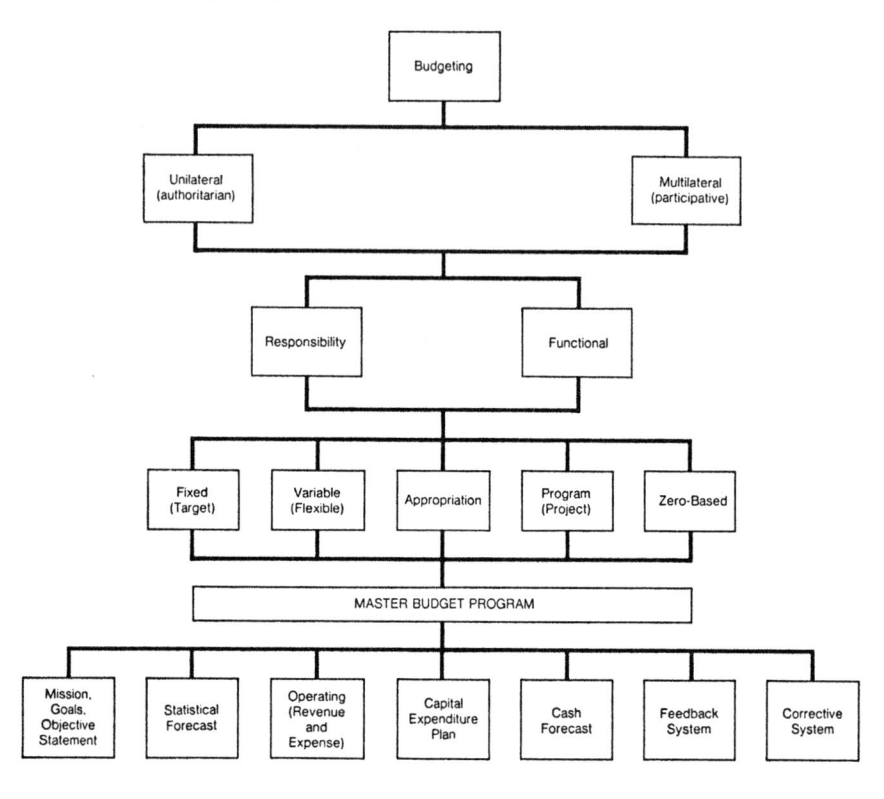

Figure 6–4 Budgeting Classification Tree

are eight basic components, as shown in Figure 6–5, that are likely to remain constant in most budgetary control systems:

- statement of purpose
- statistical forecast
- operating budget
- capital expenditure plan
- cash flow forecast
- operations
- performance evaluation and corrective measures
- plan review and adjustment

Figure 6-5 The Budgetary Control System, Memorial Hospital, Anytown, U.S.A.

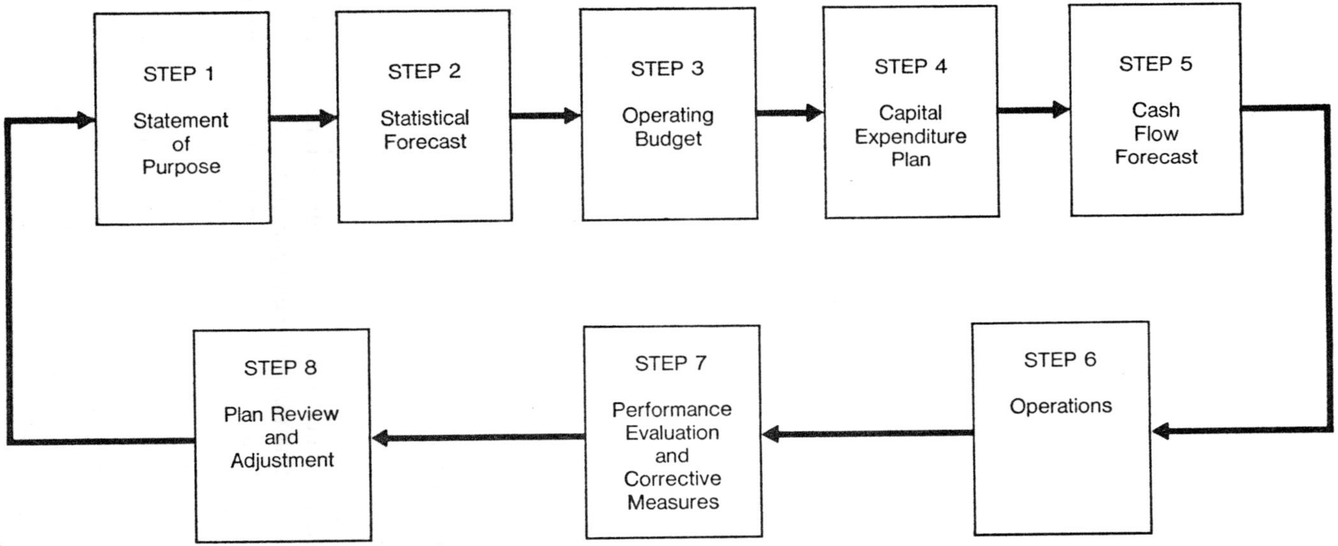

- STEP 1: Statement of Purpose
- STEP 2: Statistical Forecast
- STEP 3: Operating Budget
- STEP 4: Capital Expenditure Plan
- STEP 5: Cash Flow Forecast
- STEP 6: Operations
- STEP 7: Performance Evaluation and Corrective Measures
- STEP 8: Plan Review and Adjustment

The statement of purpose is a narrative report that identifies and quantifies the department's:

- mission
- goals and objectives
- assumptions
- strategy to be used to obtain these goals and objectives
- required resources
- standards of acceptable or expected performance

The statement of purpose requires information and involvement of top management and middle management. When the statement and standards are mutually accepted, the data are documented and subsequently serve as the foundation for all the budgets and evaluating mechanisms in the total budgetary control system.

The statistical forecast forms the basis for all financial projections. Volume or statistical forecasting is so vital to the success of any health care institution's financial plan that it is frequently referred to as the keystone because it literally ties the revenue and expense plans together.[9] The statistical forecast includes such inpatient and outpatient statistics as:

- admissions
- discharges
- preadmissions
- initial billings
- follow-up billings
- accounts in file
- patient consultations
- telephone calls
- letters typed

These, as well as many other statistics and established performance standards, are used to determine staffing requirements.

The operating budget is the statement of purpose and statistical forecast expressed in financial terms. Because the patient business services department is a cash-generating department rather than a revenue-producing center, the primary components of the department's operating budget are:

- salary and fringe benefit expenses
- nonsalary and supply expenses
- provision for depreciation

The first two expense categories represent eventual cash outflows, whereas depreciation is a noncash item which represents an accounting provision to amortize the purchase of capital assets. It is essential to separate cash and noncash items to facilitate cash flow forecasting. Essentially, the operating budget is a tool to assist management in short-term planning and control of current operating needs. It usually spans a minimum of one year.

The capital expenditure plan represents management's perception of the capital needs for a long period of time—usually a minimum of three years. A well-devised capital expenditure plan ensures that the equipment and facilities needed to support overall hospital and individual department programs will be available at the proper time. In this type of planning, cash requirements for new capital assets and the replacement of existing assets are controlled by a centralized development program. The capital expenditure plan also facilitates the establishment of priorities for asset acquisition and project selection.[10]

The cash flow forecast is a plan for projecting cash inflows and outflows and the resulting cash balances. The forecast serves as the mechanism or instrument that expresses in cash terms the operating budget and capital expenditure plan. The primary objective of the cash flow forecast is to determine whether sufficient cash resources will be available at the appropriate time to meet all the planned operating and capital cash requirements. Before the cash flow forecast can begin, the operating budget and capital expenditure plan must be completed.

All the time and resources spent in developing the above planning instruments would be futile if feedback and performance evaluation were not included in the total budgetary control system. A well-designed budgetary control system should be a self-regulating system with built-in provisions for reporting to the responsible individual actual performance as compared with the plan. The system should also require individual employees to report to the supervisor reasons for unfavorable variances and corrective measures to be taken. When performance has been evaluated and corrective measures taken, the next step is to review the original plan and make any necessary adjustments to it.

As illustrated in Figure 6–5, the budgetary control system is a never-ending cycle. A responsive budgetary control system (see Figure 6–6) is a constantly revolving cycle of:

- plan
- perform
- two-way feedback
- performance evaluation
- corrective action

Figure 6–6 Budgetary Control System

```
END Planning Cycle Here          START Planning Cycle Here
                    ┌─────────────┐
                    │   Mission   │
                    │    Goals    │
                    │  Objectives │
                    └─────────────┘
         START              END
         corrective-        corrective-action
         action cycle       here
         here

   ┌──────────────┐                    ┌──────────────┐
   │  Monitoring  │                    │  Strategies  │
   │   Feedback   │                    │  Resources   │
   │  Evaluation  │                    │  Standards   │
   │  Corrective- │                    │ Assumptions  │
   │    Action    │                    │              │
   └──────────────┘                    └──────────────┘

                    ┌──────────────┐
                    │Implementation│
                    │  Operation   │
                    └──────────────┘
```

———— Operating Cycle

- - - - Corrective-Action Cycle

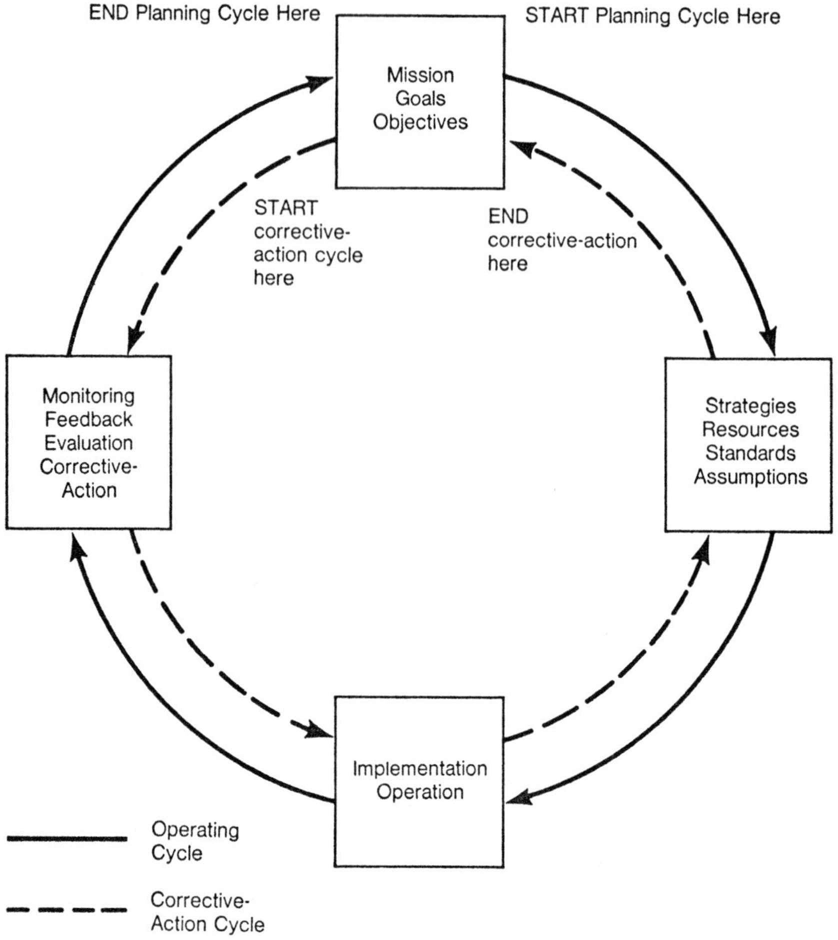

In the budgetary control system, the completion of one cycle begins another.

In short, an effective budgetary control system helps create a management style that involves all levels of the management hierarchy. It also uses the hands-on experience of each level of employee to help formulate a cohesive plan that will improve the quality as well as the quantity of work performed. However, one word of caution: the budgetary control system is not a panacea, nor does it work by itself. It not only requires constant nurturing and evaluation, but it also requires the total cooperation of all levels of people—the skilled and the nonskilled, the managers and the managed. Simply speaking, it requires dedication and commitment.

NOTES

1. Allen G. Herkimer, Jr., *Understanding Hospital Financial Management* (Germantown, Md.: Aspen Systems Corp., 1978), p. 131.
2. *The Management of Patient Account Services: Unit I—Strategy*, 6th printing (Oak Brook, Ill.: Hospital Financial Management Educational Foundation, 1979), pp. 1–26.
3. Allen G. Herkimer, Jr., *Concepts in Hospital Financial Management*, 2nd ed. (Northridge, Calif.: Alfa Associates, Inc., 1973), p. 75.
4. Peter F. Drucker, *Managing for Results* (New York: Harper & Row, 1964), p. 3.
5. Herkimer, *Understanding Hospital Financial Management*, p. 62.
6. J. Brooks Heckert and James D. Willson, *Controllership*, 2nd ed. (New York: Ronald Press Co., 1963), p. 72.
7. Herkimer, *Understanding Hospital Financial Management*, pp. 142–143.
8. Peter A. Pyhrr, *Zero-Base Budgeting* (New York: John Wiley & Sons, 1973), p. 5.
9. Herkimer, *Understanding Hospital Financial Management*, p. 103.
10. *Budgeting Manual*, 2nd ed. (Sacramento, Calif.: California Health Facilities Commission, 1977), p. 69.

Chapter 7
Application of Variable Budgeting

Variable budgeting is based on the principle of cost variability. Cost variability refers to the fact that costs can be related to work volume or output and that they are the result of two factors: (1) time, and (2) volume.

Under the principle of cost variability, costs related to activity may be classified as either fixed or variable. In reality, a third type of cost also exists—the step- or semi-variable cost (see Chapter 4). In order to classify costs in these categories, it is essential to clearly define each natural cost classification. Classification of costs for the patient business services department will be discussed later in the chapter.

In applying the variable budgeting concept to the patient business services department, it is important to remember that the degree of accuracy management requires determines how sound the eventual analysis and decision making will be. Data for managerial use must be accurate, but that requirement does not preclude the use of reasonable estimates.[1] It has been stated that judgment is approximately 80 to 85 percent of forecasting—it is an art. Sound judgment is the basis of any effective budgetary control system.

PURPOSE OF VARIABLE BUDGETING

The primary purposes of variable budgeting are to:

- assist management in controlling expenses, and
- eliminate budget variances due to volume changes.

Variable budgets provide expense information that makes it possible to compensate for differences in volume and rates. Essentially, the variable budget develops a methodology for classifying each and every expense in any department. That methodology establishes the relationship of these expense categories to the production units generated by the department.

The variable budget attempts to solve the most common problem in performance reports, that is, comparison of actual expenses with a budget allowance that is adjusted to the level of activity or output attained.[2] Variable budgets are dynamic instruments that can be quickly and automatically adjusted to any change in volume of activity.

RELATIONSHIP OF STANDARD COSTS TO VARIABLE BUDGETING

Standard costs are the building blocks of a variable budgeting control system. They are carefully developed costs established by management as desirable costs per unit of service. They are based on standards established by management for specific tasks or groups of tasks. The standards indicate the resources—labor, supplies, equipment—required to perform the tasks. Essentially, standard costs express in financial terms what specific tasks should cost per production unit. Horngren states that standard costs are often divided into three types:[3]

1. basic
2. maximum efficiency
3. attainable

Basic cost standards are unchanging standards that provide a basis for comparing actual costs. Since this type of standard is inflexible, basic cost standards are seldom used because they do not reflect market fluctuations or changes in costs and methods.

Maximum efficiency cost standards represent the absolute minimum cost possible under the best conceivable operating conditions.[4] Use of this standard is relatively limited; however, it can be used to motivate employees to achieve greater productivity. The danger is that maximum efficiency standards may, instead, discourage employees from improving productivity.

The third and most commonly used standard cost is the attainable cost. This standard tends to be less restrictive than the maximum efficiency standard because it allows for down-time and lost time. However, the attainable standard is strict enough to encourage improved productivity and to give employees a sense of achievement when they reach the standard. The major benefits of using attainable standard costs derive from the fact that they can be used to:

- develop production unit costs
- develop departmental and total hospital costs
- motivate employees

Regardless of the type of standard used, it is the bridge that allows the budget analyst to adjust a target budget to a variable budget, that is, to adjust a fixed volume departmental or unit cost to the actual volume departmental or unit cost. This capacity of cost standards is essential for effective and prudent management, especially in times in which the hospital industry is experiencing dynamic changes in use of hospital services coupled with ravaging inflation.

The variable budget control system offers management a unique tool for expense control. The basic objectives of any cost control program are to:

- control the production unit cost
- maintain or increase production per employee

The variable budget concept is designed to meet these objectives.

DEVELOPING STANDARD RATES AND COSTS

Standard rates and costs can be developed for the institution as a whole, for each department, or for individual services or items. Institutional and/or departmental standards can be developed to allow management to determine the volume of service a hospital and/or a department requires to break even as illustrated below.

Computation of Break Even Daily Census	Amount	Percent
1. Average net charge per patient day	$600	100%
2. Average variable cost per patient day	200	33⅓%
3. Contribution	$400	
4. Contribution margin		66⅔%
5. Fixed expenses per calendar day	$40,000	
6. Desired profit per calendar day	$20,000	
7. Total fixed expenses and desired profit per calendar day	$60,000	
8. Break even census per calendar day (line 7 ÷ line 3 = line 8)	150 patient days	
9. Break even net charges per calendar day (line 7 ÷ line 4 = line 9)	$90,000	

To be most effective, standard rates and costs should be developed for each revenue service, expense item, and salaried position. This enables the analyst to localize any major variance between actual performance and the standard. The development of individual standards will be discussed in more detail in the case study at the end of this chapter.

The basic formulas for developing standards are:

A. *Standard Rate Formula*

$$\frac{\text{Total revenue}}{\text{Total relevant units of service}} = \text{Standard rate}$$

B. *Standard Cost Formula*

$$\frac{\text{Total variable expense}}{\text{Total relevant units of services}} = \text{Standard cost}$$

As illustrated, standards can be developed for revenue and expenses. Generally, the term "standard rate" refers to a charge for an individual service generated by a revenue-producing department or the average rate an employee is paid per hour. The term "standard cost" refers to the amount of any specific expense–variable item per unit of service.

DEVELOPING THE VARIABLE BUDGET

The basic objectives of the variable budget concept were identified above. The fixed budget methodology is not designed to satisfy these objectives; however, the fixed budget is used as the forecast or target budget from which standard rates and costs are developed for the variable budgetary control system. The following is a step-by-step approach to developing a variable budget for the patient business services department of Memorial Hospital of Anytown, U.S.A.

Step 1. Identify the fixed salary and nonsalary expense items in the department's chart of accounts. These fixed expenses will not change within a relevant range of activity or volume, yet they are incurred no matter how many production units the department produces. It is important to note that costs identified as fixed in one department or hospital will not necessarily be fixed costs in another setting. The analyst must relate cost behavior to the specific environment. According to the chart of accounts shown in Table 7–1, the following expense items have been classified as fixed:

Fixed Expenses: Patient Business Services Department
Salaries and Wages
.01 Management and Supervision
.02 Executive Secretaries
.10 Employee Benefits—Executive

Nonsalary Expenses
.21 Dues and Subscriptions
.22 Equipment Rentals and Leases
.24 Travel
.29 Training Programs
.30 Depreciation

Step 2. In this illustration, assume that all remaining items are direct variable costs, even though some expense categories, such as salaries for the admitting, billing, and collection clerks, are in fact step-variable ex-

Table 7–1 Chart of Accounts, Memorial Hospital, Anytown, U.S.A.

Patient Business Services Department
Department Expenses
Code No.   Description
Salary and Wages
.01 Management and Supervision
.02 Executive Secretaries
.03 Admitting Clerks
.04 Billing Clerks
.05 Collection Clerks
.10 Employee Benefits—Executive
.11 Employee Benefits—Staff

Nonsalary Expenses
.21 Dues and Subscriptions
.22 Equipment Rentals and Leases
.23 Telephone
.24 Travel
.25 Postage
.26 Collection Fees
.27 Printed Forms
.28 Other Office Supplies
.29 Training Programs
.30 Depreciation

penses. (This matter will be discussed more fully later in this chapter.) The department's cost classification chart of accounts is illustrated in Table 7–2.

Step 3. Select a production unit that will represent the work performed in the department reasonably accurately. For illustration, the number of inpatient and outpatient admissions has been selected as the macro or gross departmental production unit. Selecting this unit does not preclude the use of other production units to measure individual position or expense categories. In this case, the number of admissions will be the basis for establishing departmental production and cost standards.

Step 4. Using the target or fixed budget (see Table 7–3), record these expense classifications and amounts in the appropriate location on the variable budget worksheet shown in Table 7–4.

Table 7–2 Cost Classification—Chart of Accounts, Memorial Hospital, Anytown, U.S.A.

Patient Business Services Department
Departmental Production Unit: Number of Admissions (Inpatient and Outpatient)

DEPARTMENT EXPENSES

Cost Behavior

Code No.	Description	Direct Variable Method	Step-Variable Method
Salaries and Wages			
.01	Management and Supervision	Fixed	Fixed
.02	Executive Secretaries	Fixed	Fixed
.03	Admitting Clerks	Variable	Step-Variable
.04	Billing Clerks	Variable	Step-Variable
.05	Collection Clerks	Variable	Step-Variable
.10	Employee Benefits—Management	Fixed	Fixed
.11	Employee Benefits—Staff	Variable	Step-Variable
Nonsalary Expenses			
.21	Dues and Subscriptions	Fixed	Fixed
.22	Equipment Rentals and Leases	Fixed	Fixed
.23	Telephone	Variable	Variable
.24	Travel	Fixed	Fixed
.25	Postage	Variable	Variable
.26	Collection Fees	Variable	Variable
.27	Printed Forms	Variable	Variable
.28	Other Office Supplies	Variable	Variable
.29	Training Programs	Fixed	Fixed
.30	Depreciation	Fixed	Fixed

Application of Variable Budgeting 139

Table 7–3 Target or Fixed Budget

Memorial Hospital, Anytown, U.S.A.
Patient Business Services Department
Target or Fixed Budget
For the Fiscal Year Ending September 30, 19x1

	Total Amount	Hours
Volume		
Number of Admissions:		
Inpatient	6,738	
Outpatient	31,025	
Total Admissions	37,763	
Salaries and Wages		
Management and Supervision	$ 55,000	4,160
Executive Secretaries	18,000	2,080
Admitting Clerks	85,000	17,680
Billing Clerks	60,000	12,480
Collection Clerks	48,000	8,320
Employee Benefits—Management	18,250	n/a
Employee Benefits—Staff	48,250	n/a
Total Salaries and Wages	$332,500	44,720
Nonsalary Expenses		
Dues and Subscriptions	$ 1,000	
Equipment Rentals and Leases	21,600	
Telephone	10,800	
Travel	6,000	
Postage	32,000	
Collection Fees	180,000	
Printed Forms	75,500	
Other Office Supplies	38,000	
Training Programs	6,000	
Depreciation	12,000	
Total Nonsalary Expenses	$382,900	
Total Expenses	$715,400	

Step 5. Record the target budget hours in the appropriate spaces in the variable budget worksheet.

Step 6. Using the total volume of production units (column 5, line 7, in Table 7–4), compute the variable expense standard for each variable item.

Table 7-4 Variable Budget Worksheet

Memorial Hospital, Anytown, U.S.A.
Variable Budget Worksheet
For the Fiscal Year Ending September 30, 19x1

Department: Patient Business Services
Production Unit: Number of Admissions (Inpatient and Outpatient)

HOURS — TARGET BUDGET			ACCOUNT DESCRIPTION	EXPENSES — TARGET BUDGET		
Fixed (1)	Variable (2)	Variable Production Standard (3)	(4)	Fixed (5)	Variable (6)	Variable Expense Standard (7)
			Salaries and Wages			
4,160		n/a	1. (a) Management & Supervision	55,000		n/a
2,080		n/a	(b) Executive Secretaries	18,000		n/a
	17,680	2.14	(c) Admitting Clerks		85,000	2.25
	12,480	3.03	(d) Billing Clerks		60,000	1.59
	8,320	4.54	(e) Collection Clerks		48,000	1.27
			(f) Employee Benefits—Management			n/a
			(g) Employee Benefits—Staff	18,250	48,250	n/a
6,240	38,480	0.98	2. Total Salaries & Wages	91,250	241,250	6.39

Application of Variable Budgeting   141

HOURS			EXPENSES		
TARGET BUDGET		ACCOUNT DESCRIPTION (4)	TARGET BUDGET		
Fixed (1)	Variable (2)	Variable Production Standard (3)		Fixed (5)	Variable (6)	Variable Expense Standard (7)

Fixed (1)	Variable (2)	Variable Production Standard (3)	ACCOUNT DESCRIPTION (4)	Fixed (5)	Variable (6)	Variable Expense Standard (7)
		Computation of Variable Standard Hourly Rates	Nonsalary Expenses			
			3. (a) Dues & Subscriptions	1,000		n/a
			(b) Equipment Rentals & Leases	21,600		n/a
		Position St. Hr. Rate	(c) Telephone		10,800	.29
		Admitting Clerks 4.81	(d) Travel	6,000		n/a
		Billing Clerks 4.81	(e) Postage		32,000	.85
		Collection Clerks 5.77	(f) Collection Fees		180,000	4.76
		Employee Benefits 1.25	(g) Printed Forms		75,500	2.00
		Total 6.27	(h) Other Office Supplies		38,000	1.00
		Formula:	(i) Training Programs	6,000		n/a
		Total Salary Expense (col. 6)	(j) Depreciation	12,000		n/a
		Total Hours (col. 2)	4. Total Nonsalary Expenses	46,600	336,300	8.90
		= Variable Standard Hourly Rate				
			5. Grand Total Expenses	137,850	577,550	
			Number of Admissions (Volume)			
			6. (a) Inpatient	6,738		
			(b) Outpatient	31,025		
			7. Total Admissions	37,763		

For example:

$$\frac{\text{Total admitting clerk expense (column 6, line 1(c))}}{\text{Total relevant number of admissions (column 5, line 7)}} = \text{Standard costs per admission}$$

or

$$\frac{\$85,000}{37,763} = \$2.25$$

and record in column 7, line 1(c).

Step 7. Using the total volume of production units (column 5, line 7, in Table 7–4), compute the variable production standards for each variable salary and wage expense position as follows:

$$\frac{\text{Total number of admissions (column 5, line 7)}}{\text{Total relevant admitting clerk hours (column 2, line 1(c))}} = \text{Variable production standard}$$

or

$$\frac{37,763}{17,680} = 2.14 \text{ admissions per hour}$$

and record in column 3, line 1(c).

When Step 7 has been completed, variable production standards have been developed for each position and for the department as follows:

Salaries and Wages	*Variable Production Standard*
Admitting Clerks	2.14 admissions per hour
Billing Clerks	3.03 admissions per hour
Collection Clerks	4.54 admissions per hour
Total Variable Positions	0.98 admissions per hour

Variable expense (costs) standards have also been developed for each expense category and for the department as follows:

Salaries and Wages	Variable Standard Cost
Admitting Clerks	$2.25 per admission
Billing Clerks	1.59 per admission
Collection Clerks	1.27 per admission
Employee Benefits—Staff	1.28 per admission
Total Salaries and Wages	$6.39 per admission

Nonsalary Expenses	Variable Standard Cost
Telephone	$0.29 per admission
Postage	9.85 per admission
Collection Fees	4.75 per admission
Printed Forms	2.00 per admission
Other Office Supplies	1.00 per admission
Total Nonsalary Expenses	$8.90 per admission

These standards will remain relatively consistent throughout the budget year, barring any major changes in systems or costs, and will be used to develop the direct-variable control budgets. Control budgets are budgets that show targeted fixed expense levels with direct-variable expense categories adjusted according to the actual work volume. The direct-variable expense categories are adjusted by multiplying standard rates by actual volume of work performed. The variable budget eliminates performance variances due to volume changes. The development and use of control budgets will be discussed in more detail later in this chapter.

For further illustration of the application of the variable budget, assume that during the course of the year, the patient business services department at Memorial Hospital experienced a 2,873 decrease in the amount of budgeted admissions from 37,763 to 34,890. Assume further that the patient account manager retained the variable staff level budgeted on the basis of a higher volume of work. Table 7–5 is a comparative analysis of the original target (fixed volume) budget and the actual performance. When the patient account manager initially reviews this analysis (see summary below), he/she would be very pleased with department performance because there is a favorable variance of $17,500 for nonsalary expense, and salary and wage expense is exactly as budgeted.

	Actual	Budget	Variance
Total salaries and wages	$332,500	$332,500	$ -0-
Total nonsalary expenses	365,400	382,900	17,500
Total expenses	$697,900	$715,400	$17,500

144 PATIENT ACCOUNT MANAGEMENT

Table 7-5 Comparative Analysis of Fixed Target Budget to Actual Performance

Memorial Hospital, Anytown, U.S.A.
Patient Business Services Department
Comparative Analysis of Fixed Target Budget to Actual Performance
For the Fiscal Year Ending September 30, 19x1

	Actual	Budget	Volume Fav. (Unfav.)
Salaries and Wages			
Management and Supervision	$56,000	$55,000	$(1,000)
Executive Secretaries	18,000	18,000	-0-
Admitting Clerks	83,000	85,000	2,000
Billing Clerks	62,000	60,000	(2,000)
Collection Clerks	47,000	48,000	1,000
Employee Benefits—Management	19,250	18,250	(1,000)
Employee Benefits—Staff	47,250	48,250	1,000
Total Salaries and Wages	$332,500	$332,500	-0-
Nonsalary Expenses			
Dues and Subscriptions	$ 900	$ 1,000	$ 100
Equipment Rental and Leases	21,600	21,600	-0-
Telephone	9,400	10,800	1,400
Travel	5,000	6,000	1,000
Postage	30,000	32,000	2,000
Collection Fees	170,000	180,000	10,000
Printed Forms	74,000	75,500	1,500
Other Office Supplies	36,500	38,000	1,500
Training Programs	6,000	6,000	-0-
Depreciation	12,000	12,000	-0-
Total Nonsalary Expenses	$365,400	$382,900	$17,500
Total Expenses	$697,900	$715,400	$17,500

However, the analysis must be extended to an evaluation of volume and paid hours. These data are analyzed and compared in Table 7-6. The first indication of any problem is the unfavorable variance of 2,873 in the number of admissions. This represents a 7.6 percent decrease in work volume. The second indication of a possible problem is the relatively small favorable decrease of 350 variable hours. This decrease, actually 1.0 percent, is small compared to the 7.6 percent decrease in work volume. At this point, a control budget must be developed to allow for these volume variances and to adjust variable expenses to match actual volume of work.

Application of Variable Budgeting   145

Table 7-6 Comparative Analysis of Volume and Variable Paid Hours

Memorial Hospital, Anytown, U.S.A.
Patient Business Services Department
Comparative Analysis of Volume to Variable Paid Hours
For the Fiscal Year Ending September 30, 19x1

	Actual	Budget	Variance Fav. (Unfav.)
Volume			
Number of Admissions:			
Inpatient	6,280	6,738	(458)
Outpatient	28,610	31,025	(2,415)
Total Admissions	34,890	37,763	(2,873)
Variable Paid Hours			
Admitting Clerks	17,500	17,680	180
Billing Clerks	12,480	12,480	-0-
Collection Clerks	8,150	8,320	170
Total Variable Paid Hours	38,130	38,480	350

DEVELOPING THE DIRECT-VARIABLE CONTROL BUDGET

A step-by-step approach to developing a direct-variable control budget is presented below. This control budget uses the variable standard rates developed for the target budget and adjusts the department's total variable expenses according to the actual volume of work (see Table 7-7).

Step 1. Record actual performance, that is, 34,890 admissions, in the control budget as the volume of work.

Step 2. Separate fixed expenses into two categories: (1) salaries and wages, and (2) nonsalary expenses. Record the exact amount of each expense as it was projected in the target budget.

Step 3. Record the standard rates developed in the variable budget worksheet (Table 7-4, page 140) in the appropriate column. Multiply these rates by the actual volume of work (34,890 admissions). For example:

Standard rate for admitting clerks = $2.25 per admission

Volume × Rate = Total control budget variable cost
or
34,890 × $2.25 = $78,503

Table 7-7 Comparative Analysis of Variable Control Budget to Actual Performance

Memorial Hospital, Anytown, U.S.A.
Patient Business Services Department
Comparative Analysis of Variable Control Budget to Actual Performance

	Standard Cost Per Admission	Control Budget	Actual	Variance Fav. (Unfav.)
Volume				
Number of Admissions		34,890	34,890	-0-
Fixed Expenses				
Salaries and Wages				
Management and Supervision		$ 55,000	$ 56,000	$ (1,000)
Executive Secretaries		18,000	18,000	-0-
Employee Benefits—Management		18,250	19,250	(1,000)
Total Fixed Salaries and Wages		$ 91,250	$ 93,250	$ (2,000)
Nonsalary Expenses				
Dues and Subscriptions		$ 1,000	$ 900	$ 100
Equipment Rental and Leases		21,600	21,600	-0-
Travel		6,000	5,000	1,000
Training Programs		6,000	6,000	-0-
Depreciation		12,000	12,000	-0-
Total Fixed Nonsalary Expenses		$ 46,600	$ 45,500	$ 1,100
Total Fixed Expenses		$137,850	$138,750	$ (900)
Variable Expenses				
Salaries and Wages				
Admitting Clerks	$2.25	$ 78,503	$ 83,000	$ (4,497)
Billing Clerks	1.59	55,475	62,000	(6,525)
Collection Clerks	1.27	44,310	47,000	(2,690)
Employee Benefits—Staff	1.28	44,659	47,250	(2,591)
Total Variable Salaries and Wages	$6.27	$222,947	$239,250	$(16,303)
Nonsalary Expenses				
Telephone	$ .29	$ 10.118	$ 9,400	$ 718
Postage	.85	29,657	30,000	(343)
Collection Fees	4.76	166,076	170,000	(3,924)
Printed Forms	2.00	69,980	74,000	(4,220)
Other Office Supplies	1.00	34,890	36,500	(1,610)
Total Variable Nonsalary Expenses	$8.90	$310,521	$319,900	$ (9,379)
Total Variable Expenses	$15.29	$533,468	$559,150	$(25,682)
Total Fixed and Variable Expenses		$671,318	$697,900	$(26,582)

Table 7-8 Comparative Summary Analysis

Memorial Hospital, Anytown, U.S.A.
Patient Business Services Department
Comparative Summary Analysis of Target and
Variable Control Budget to Actual Performance
For the Fiscal Year Ending September 30, 19x1

	Target	Control	Actual
Volume			
Number of Admissions	37,763	34,890	34,890
Fixed Expenses			
Salaries and Wages	$ 91,250	$ 91,250	$ 93,250
Nonsalary Expenses	46,600	46,600	45,500
Total Fixed Expenses	$137,850	$137,850	$138,750
Variable Expenses			
Salaries and Wages	$241,250	$222,947	$239,250
Nonsalary Expenses	336,300	310,521	319,900
Total Variable Expenses	$577,550	$533,468	$559,150
Total Fixed and Variable Expenses	$715,400	$671,318	$697,900

Step 4. Record the actual fixed and variable performance on the proper line in the proper column. Adjust the subtotals and totals as identified in Table 7-7.

A comparative summary of the data in the target and variable control budgets and actual performance is illustrated in Table 7-8. The comparison of the total target budget of $715,400 to total actual performance of $697,900 indicates a "favorable" variance of $17,500. However, this comparison does not take into consideration the 2,873 "unfavorable" variances from the target budget's volume forecast of 37,763 to the actual volume of 34,890. The variable budget makes provision for this volume variance and thus identifies a $26,582 "unfavorable" variance from the control budget's total of $671,318 to the actual performance total of $697,900.

ANALYSIS OF SALARY BUDGET VARIANCES

The next series of steps will indicate how specific favorable and unfavorable variances between actual performance and the control budget are analyzed. Analysis of specific budget variances in the fixed cost category is relatively simple. These variances may be summarized as follows:

	Budget Variances	
Account Description	Favorable	Unfavorable
Fixed Salaries and Wages		
Management and Supervisory		$1,000
Employee Benefits—Management		$1,000
Fixed Nonsalary Expenses		
Dues and Subscriptions	$ 100	
Travel	1,000	
Total Fixed Variances	$1,100	$2,000

The patient account manager should be ready to explain not only the unfavorable variances but also the favorable variances.

Variable budget variances are generally described as either efficiency variances or rate variances. The efficiency variance attaches a dollar amount to the difference between the number of hours budgeted for a given task and the number of hours actually required to perform it. The formula for calculating the efficiency variance is:

Efficiency variance = (Budget hours − Actual hours) ×

Standard rate

or

Difference in hours ×

Standard rate

For example: *Admitting clerks*

Target budget	17,680 hours
Actual performance	17,500 hours
Variance	180 hours (unfavorable)
Standard rate	$4.81

Efficiency variance = (17,680 − 17,500) × $4.81

= 180 × $4.81

= $8.66 (unfavorable)

The rate variance is the difference between the standard rate and the actual rate times the actual volume. The formula for calculating the rate variance is:

Rate variance = (Standard rate − Actual rate) × Actual volume

For example: *Admitting clerks*

	Target	Actual
Total expenses	$85,000	$83,000
Total hours	17,680	17,500
Average hourly rate	$4.81	$4.74

Rate variance = ($4.81 − $4.74) × 34,890

= $0.07 × 34,890

= $244 (favorable)

Table 7–9 shows the computation and analysis of efficiency and rate variances for each of the variable positions in the patient business services department. The variances shown in Table 7–9 are summarized as follows:

Position	Efficiency	Rate	Total
Admitting Clerks	$866	$1,225	$2,091
Billing Clerks	None	(1,997)	(1,997)
Collection Clerks	981	None	981
Employee Benefits—Staff	438	381	819
Total	$2,285	$ (391)	$1,894

Variance—Favorable (Unfavorable)

By exceeding their original targeted performance, the admitting and collection clerks experienced a total favorable variance of $2,285. The billing clerks, on the other hand, performed just as efficiently as they had been targeted to do. However, because the billing clerks were paid an average of $0.16 per hour more than had originally been budgeted, there was an unfavorable variance of $1,997 in their wages. Conversely, the admitting clerks' average hourly wage was $0.07 less than the target budget amount, resulting in a favorable variance of $1,225.

In this exercise, each position was analyzed, and corresponding efficiency and rate variances were computed for the position. The patient account

Table 7-9 Computation and Analysis of Variances of Variable Salary and Wage Expenses

Memorial Hospital, Anytown, U.S.A.
Patient Business Services Department
Computation and Analysis of Variances of Variable
Salaries and Wage Expenses
For the Fiscal Year Ending September 30, 19x1

Description	Admitting Clerks	Billing Clerks	Collection Clerks	Employee Benefits —Staff	Total
I. *Target Standard*					
1. Standard Hourly Rate	$ 4.81	$ 4.81	$ 5.77	$ 1.25	
2. Standard Hours	17,680	12,480	8,320	38,480	
3. Target budget (line 1 × line 2 = line 3)	$85,000	$60,000	$48,000	$48,250	
II. *Control Standard*					
4. Standard Hourly Rate (line 1)	$ 4.81	$ 4.81	$ 5.77	$ 1.25	
5. Actual Hours	17,500	12,480	8,150	38,130	
6. Control Standard (line 4 × line 5 = line 6)	$84,175	$60,029	$47,026	$47,663	
III. *Actual Performance*					
7. Actual Hourly Rate	$ 4.74	$ 4.97	$ 5.77	$ 1.24	
8. Actual Hours (line 5)	17,500	12,480	8,150	38,130	
9. Actual Performance (line 7 × line 8 = line 9)	$83,000	$62,000	$47,000	$47,250	

IV. Efficiency Variance

10. Standard Hours (line 2)	17,680	12,480	38,480
11. Actual Hours (line 5)	17,500	12,480	38,130
12. Hour Variance	180	None	350
(line 10 − line 11 = line 12)	Favorable		Favorable
13. Standard Hourly Rate	$ 4.81	$ 4.81	$ 1.25
14. Efficiency Variance	$ 866	None	$ 438	$2,285
(line 12 × line 13 = line 14)	Favorable		Favorable	Favorable

V. Rate Variance

15. Actual Hours (line 5)	17,500	12,480	38,130
16. Actual Hourly Rate (line 7)	$ 4.74	$ 4.74	$ 1.24
17. Standard Hourly Rate (line 1)	$ 4.81	$ 4.81	$ 1.25
18. Hourly Rate Variance	$ .07	$ .16	$ .01
(line 16 − line 17 = line 18)	Favorable	Unfavorable	Favorable
19. Rate Variance	$ 1,225	$ 1,997	$ 381	$ 391
(line 15 × line 18 = line 19)	Favorable	Unfavorable	Favorable	Unfavorable

VI.
20. Net Total Variances $ 2,091 $ 1,997 $ 819 $1,894
   (line 14 + line 18 = line 19)   Favorable   Unfavorable   Favorable   Favorable

VII. Proof

21. Target Budget (line 3)	$85,000	$60,000	$48,250	$48,250
22. Actual Performance (line 9)	$83,000	$62,000	$47,000	$47,250
23. Variance Target to Actual	$ 2,000	$ 2,000	$ 1,000	$2,000
(line 21 − line 22 = line 23)	Favorable	Unfavorable	Favorable	Favorable

NOTE: Differences between net total variances (line 20) and variance between target and actual (line 23) is due to rounding off all rates and totals to the nearest dollar or 100th of dollar.

manager could use the department averages to compute these variances in the following manner:

I. *Efficiency variance*

1. Standard hours — 38,480
2. Actual hours — 38,130
3. Hourly variance — 350 (favorable)
   (line 1 − line 2 = line 3)
4. Standard hourly rate — $6.27
   ($241,250 ÷ 38,480)
5. Efficiency variance — $2,195 (favorable)
   (line 3 × line 4 = line 5)

II. *Rate variance*

6. Actual hours — 38,130
7. Actual hourly rate — $6.27
   ($239,250 ÷ 38,130 hours)
8. Standard hourly rate — $6.27
9. Hourly rate variance — None
   (line 7 − line 8 = line 9)
10. Rate variance — None
    (line 6 × line 9 = line 10)
11. Net total variance — $2,195 (favorable)
    (line 5 + line 10 = line 11)

These two methods of analyzing variances may be compared in the following manner:

	Position by position	*Average position*
Efficiency variance	$2,285	$2,195 (favorable)
Rate variance	(391)	None
Net total variance	$1,894	$2,195

These differences represent less than one percent of the total variable salary and wage expense. They are probably due to rounding off totals and rates to the nearest dollar or hundredths of a dollar.

ANALYSIS OF NONSALARY EXPENSE VARIANCES

Usage variances and rate variances are two commonly used methods of analyzing the differences between budgeted and actual performance for nonsalary expenses. The usage variance is computed by multiplying the standard rate by the difference between the actual volume and the target volume. The formula is:

Usage variance = (Target volume − Actual volume) × Standard rate

For example: Telephone   = (37,763 − 34,890) × $0.29
               Usage variance   = 2,873 × $0.29
                                 = $833 favorable

This amount represents the savings experienced due to a lower volume of service.

The rate variance represents the favorable or unfavorable variance costs experienced when the actual rate differs from the target budget. The formula for the variance is:

Rate variance = (Standard unit cost − Actual unit cost) × Actual volume

For example: Telephone
               Rate variance   = ($0.29 − $0.27) × 34,890
                               = $0.02 × 34,890
                               = $698 favorable

As is the case with salary and wage expense, nonsalary expense variances can be analyzed either by individual item, as in Table 7–10, or as a composite of all variable expenses:

I. *Usage variance*
   1. Target volume   37,763
   2. Actual volume   34,890
   3. Volume variance   3,873
      (line 1 − line 2 = line 3)
   4. Standard unit cost $8.90
   5. Usage variance $25,570 (favorable)
      (line 3 × line 4 = line 5)

II. *Rate variance*
    6. Standard unit cost $8.90
    7. Actual unit cost $9.17
    8. Unit cost variance $0.27
       (line 6 − line 7 = line 8)
    9. Actual volume   34,890
    10. Rate variance $9,420 (unfavorable)
        (line 8 × line 9 = line 10)

Table 7-10 Computation and Analysis of Variances of Variable Nonsalary Expenses

Memorial Hospital, Anytown, U.S.A.
Patient Business Services Department
Computation and Analysis of Variances of Variable Nonsalary Expenses
For the Fiscal Year Ending September 30, 19x1

Description	Telephone	Postage	Collection Fees	Printed Forms	Other Office Supplies	Total
I. *Target Standard*						
1. Target Volume	37,763	37,763	37,763	37,763	37,763	
2. Standard Unit Cost	$ .29	$ .85	$ 4.76	$ 2.00	$ 1.00	
3. Target Budget (line 1 × line 2 = line 3)	$10,800	$32,000	$180,000	$75,500	$38,000	
II. *Control Standard*						
4. Actual Volume	34,890	34,890	34,890	34,890	34,890	
5. Standard Unit Cost	$ .29	$ .85	$ 4.76	$ 2.00	$ 1.00	
6. Control Cost (line 4 × line 5 = line 6)	$10,118	$29,657	$166,076	$69,780	$34,890	
III. *Actual Performance*						
7. Actual Volume	34,890	34,890	34,890	34,890	34,890	
8. Actual Unit Cost	$ .27	$ .86	$ 4.87	$ 2.12	$ 1.05	
9. Actual Total Cost (line 7 × line 8 = line 9)	$ 9,400	$30,000	$170,000	$74,000	$36,500	

Application of Variable Budgeting

IV.	*Usage Variance*				
10.	Target Volume	37,763	37,763	37,763	37,763
11.	Actual Volume	34,890	34,890	34,890	34,890
12.	Volume Variance (line 10 − line 11 = line 12)	2,873 (favorable)	2,873 (favorable)	2,873 (favorable)	2,873 (favorable)
13.	Standard Unit Cost	$ .29	$ .85	$ 4.76	$ 2.00	$ 1.00
14.	Usage Variance (line 12 × line 13 = line 14)	$ 833 (favorable)	$ 2,442 (favorable)	$ 13,675 (favorable)	$ 5,746 (favorable)	$ 2,873 (favorable)	$25,569 (favorable)
V.	*Rate Variance*				
15.	Standard Unit Cost	$ .29	$ .85	$ 4.76	$ 2.00	$ 1.00
16.	Actual Unit Cost	$ .27	$ .86	$ 4.87	$ 2.12	$ 1.05
17.	Unit Cost Variance (line 15 − line 16 = line 17)	$ .02 (favorable)	$ .01 (unfavorable)	$ .11 (unfavorable)	$ .12 (unfavorable)	$ .05 (unfavorable)
18.	Actual Volume	34,890	34,890	34,890	34,890	34,890
19.	Rate Variance (line 17 × line 18 = line 19)	$ 698 (favorable)	$ 349 (unfavorable)	$ 3,838 (unfavorable)	$ 4,187 (unfavorable)	$ 1,745 (unfavorable)	$ 9,421 (unfavorable)
VI.	*Net Total Variance* (line 14 + line 19 = line 20)	$ 1,531 (favorable)	$ 2,093 (unfavorable)	$ 9,832 (favorable)	$ 1,559 (favorable)	$ 1,128 (unfavorable)	$16,148 (favorable)
VII.	*Proof*				
21.	Target Budget	$10,800	$32,000	$180,000	$75,000	$38,000
22.	Actual Total Costs	$ 9,400	$30,000	$170,000	$74,000	$36,500
23.	Variance—Target to Actual (line 21 − line 22 = line 23)	$ 1,400 (favorable)	$ 2,000 (favorable)	$ 10,000 (favorable)	$ 1,000 (favorable)	$ 1,500 (favorable)	$15,900 (favorable)

NOTE: Differences between Net Total Variances (line 20) and variance between target and actual (line 23) is due to rounding off all rates and totals to the nearest dollar or 100th of dollar; there is no substantial difference.

Figure 7-1 Step-Variable Cost Behavior, Memorial Hospital, Anytown, U.S.A.

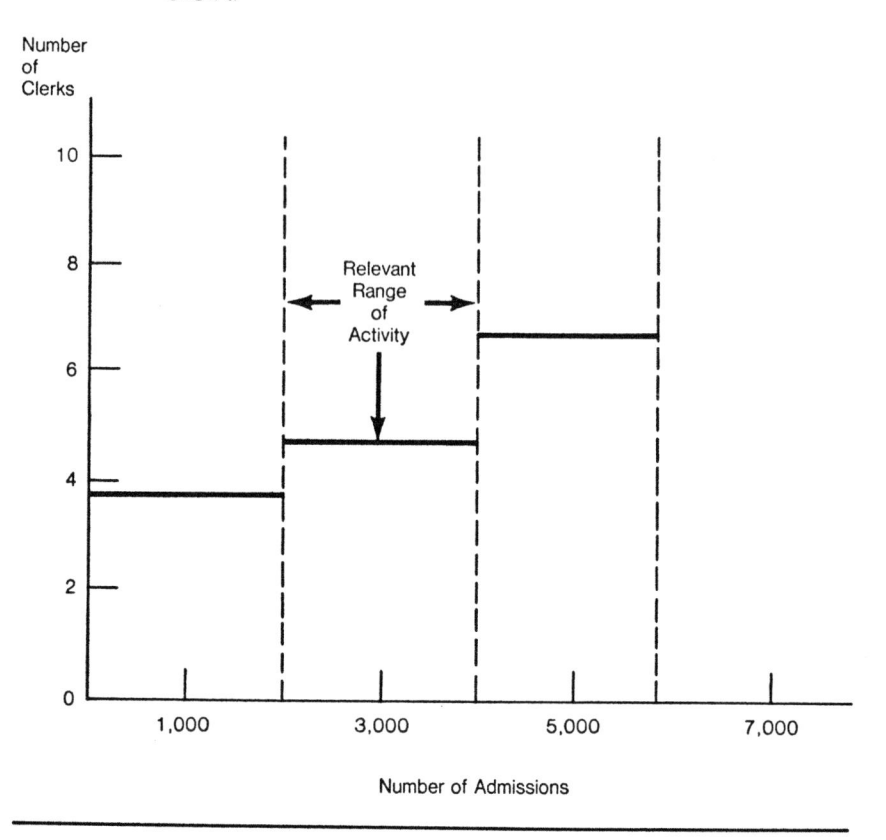

III. *Net total variance*
(line 5 + line 10 = line 11) $16,150 (favorable)

When wage and salary expenses are analyzed using these two methods, the minimal differences that result are due to the rounding off of the numbers used. The important point is that the analyst can find out why variances occurred. These examples illustrate the direct variable application of the variable budget concept. In other words, all variable expenses have been adjusted in direct proportion to the volume of work. It may be said, with some justification, that variable salary and wage expense cannot be adjusted in direct proportion to the volume of work. The patient account manager will not hire an additional admitting clerk just because admissions increase by 20, nor will he/she release one clerk just because admissions

Figure 7-2 Direct Variable Cost Behavior, Memorial Hospital, Anytown, U.S.A.

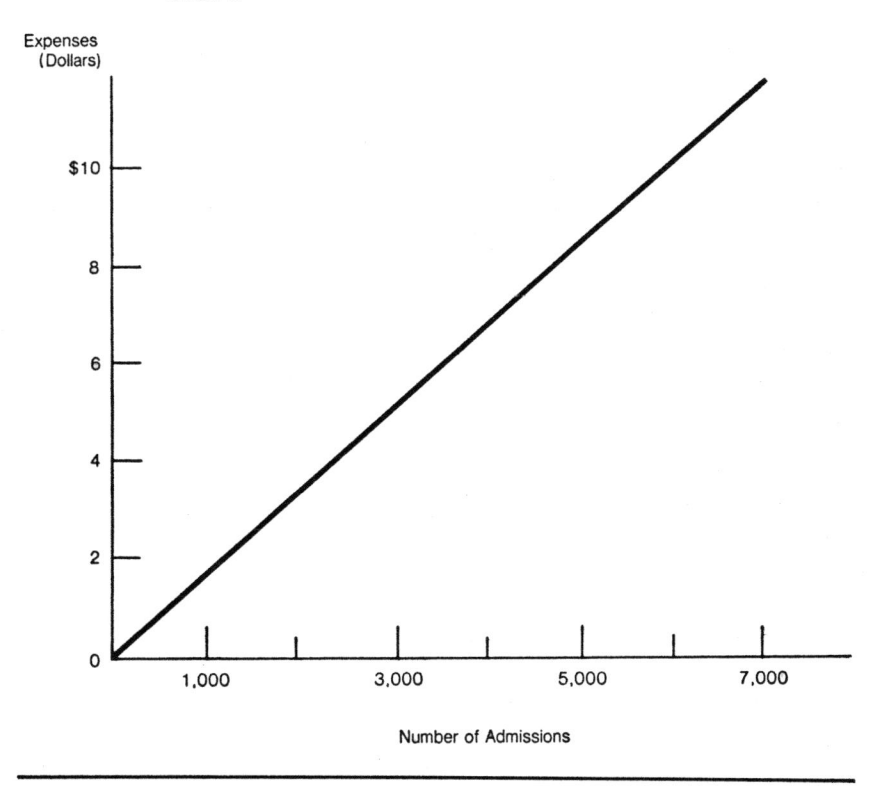

drop by 20. As noted earlier in this book, there is a certain amount of elasticity in any staff over a relevant period of time. This elasticity tends to create certain plateaus in the staffing of the patient business services department. These plateaus, in turn, result in a step-variable condition which is a lag factor for the department to adjust to volume changes.

STEP-VARIABLE STAFFING AND VARIANCE ANALYSIS

Step-variable expenses are costs that change abruptly at intervals of activity because they are experienced in indivisible chunks.[5] In practice, most clerks often experience uneven workloads. The staff elasticity factor means that the clerks can maintain an intensive or leisurely work pace for long periods of time or for a relevant range of activity as illustrated in Figure 7-1. On the other hand, expenses such as office supplies and forms

158 PATIENT ACCOUNT MANAGEMENT

Table 7–11 Computation of Step-Variable Adjustment to Actual Volume of Work

Memorial Hospital, Anytown, U.S.A.
Patient Business Services Department
Computation of Step-Variable Adjustment to Actual Volume of Work
For the Fiscal Year Ending September 30, 19x1

Description	Admitting Clerks	Billing Clerks	Collection Clerks	Employee Benefits—Staff	Total
1. Target Budget Volume	37,763	37,763	37,763	37,763	37,763
2. Budget Hours (Paid)	17,680	12,480	8,320	38,480	38,480
3. Units per Paid (line 1 ÷ line 2 = line 3)	2.14	3.03	4.54	0.98	0.98
4. Average Hours per Week	40	40	40	40	40
5. Average Weeks per Year	52	52	52	52	52
6. Average Hours per Year (line 4 × line 5 = line 6)	2,080	2,080	2,080	2,080	2,080
7. Average Annual Production (line 3 × line 6 = line 7)	4,451	6,302	9,443	2,038	2,038
8. Budget Volume (line 1)	37,763	37,763	37,763	37,763	37,763
9. Actual Volume	34,890	34,890	34,890	34,890	34,890
10. Volume Variance (line 8 − line 9 = line 10)	2,873	2,873	2,873	2,873	2,873
11. Average Annual Production (line 7) ÷ (Length of Step-Variable)	4,451	6,302	9,443	2,038	2,038
12. Average Number of Steps (line 10 ÷ line 11 = line 12)	0.65	0.46	0.30	1.41	1.41
13. Standard Hourly Wage	$ 4.81	$ 4.81	$ 5.77	$ 1.25	$ 6.27
14. Average Cost per Step (line 6 × line 13 = line 14)	$10,005	$10,005	$12,002	$2,600	$13,042
15. Step-Variable Adjustment (line 12 × line 14 = line 15)	None	None	None	$2,600	$13,042
				(Unfavorable)	(Unfavorable)

Note: Use only whole numbers on line 12.

tend to vary in direct proportion to the actual volume of work as illustrated in Figure 7–2. Table 7–11 is an example of how step-variable expense analysis can be used to analyze budget variances. The step-variable adjustment for each variable position, as computed in Table 7–11, by individual position, is:

Position	Step-Variable Adjustment
Admitting Clerks	None
Billing Clerks	None
Collection Clerks	None
Employee Benefits—Staff	$2,600
Total Step-Variable Adjustment	$2,600 (unfavorable)

When the step-variable adjustment is computed in the aggregate, there is a total unfavorable adjustment of $13,042.

The step-variable adjustment is included in the step-variable control budget and compared to actual performance (see Table 7–12). In this example, the total unfavorable step-variable variance of $13,042 is used to

Table 7–12 Comparative Analysis of Step-Variable Budget to Actual Performance

Memorial Hospital, Anytown, U.S.A.
Patient Business Services Department
Comparative Analysis of Step-Variable Budget to Actual Performance
For the Fiscal Year Ending September 30, 19x1

Description	Control Budget	Actual	Variance Fav (Unfav)
Volume			
Number of Admissions	34,890	34,890	-0-
Fixed Expenses			
Salaries and Wages	$ 91,250	$ 93,250	$ (2,000)
Nonsalary Expenses	46,600	45,500	1,100
Total Fixed Expenses	$137,850	$138,750	$ (900)
Variable Expenses			
Salaries and Wages	$228,208	$238,250	$(11,042)
Nonsalary Expenses	310,521	319,900	(9,379)
Total Variable Expenses	$538,729	$559,150	$(20,421)
Total Fixed and Variable Expenses	$676,579	$697,900	$(21,321)

160 PATIENT ACCOUNT MANAGEMENT

Table 7–13 Comparative Summary Analysis

Memorial Hospital, Anytown, U.S.A.
Patient Business Services Department
Comparative Summary Analysis of Actual Performance to Target Direct Variable and
Step-Variable Control Budgets
For the Fiscal Year Ending September 30, 19x1

Description	Actual Performance	Target Budget	Direct Variable Control Budget	Step-Variable Control Budget
Volume				
Number of Admissions	34,890	37,763	34,890	34,890
Fixed Expenses				
Salaries and Wages	$ 93,250	$ 91,250	$ 91,250	$ 91,250
Nonsalary Expenses	45,500	46,600	46,600	46,600
Total Fixed Expenses	$138,750	$137,850	$137,850	$137,850
Variable Expenses				
Salaries and Wages	$239,250	$241,250	$222,947	$228,208
Nonsalary Expenses	319,900	336,300	310,521	310,521
Total Variable Expenses	$559,150	$577,550	$533,468	$538,729
Total Fixed and Variable Expenses	$697,900	$715,400	$671,318	$676,579

arrive at the summary adjusted step-variable salary and wage control total as follows:

Original target budget salary and wage expense Variable expense	$241,250
Less: unfavorable step-variable	13,042
Adjusted step-variable salary and wage expense	$228,208

The summary analysis presented in Table 7–13 compares actual performance, the target budget, the direct variable control budget, and the step-variable control budget. In all cases, fixed expenses are the same in all budgets, while variable expenses are adjusted according to the actual volume. Nonsalary expenses are adjusted to $310,521 in each of the variable control budgets. The major differences are in the variable salary and wage expenses as summarized below:

Description	Actual	Budget	Variance
Target budget	$239,250	$241,250	$ (2,000)
Direct-variable budget	$239,250	$222,947	$(16,303)
Step-variable budget	$239,250	$228,208	$(11,042)

In summary, there is no precise or perfect method of establishing a variable budgeting system. What needs to be done is to design a system that best fits the needs of the individual department or hospital. The patient account manager and his/her supervisors and subordinates should agree on which costs are fixed, direct variable, or step-variable. Once that has been accomplished, it is possible to design management reports that will produce the desired results. Certainly, a variable budgeting control system will provide management with a more realistic report for cost control and effectiveness.

NOTES

1. Glenn A. Welsch, *Budgeting: Profit Planning and Control* (Englewood Cliffs, N.J.: Prentice-Hall, Inc., 1971), p. 310.
2. Ibid., p. 307.
3. Charles T. Horngren, *Cost Accounting: A Managerial Emphasis*, 3rd ed. (Englewood Cliffs, N.J.: Prentice-Hall, Inc., 1972), p. 187.
4. Ibid., p. 185.
5. Charles T. Horngren, *Accounting for Management Control: An Introduction* (Englewood Cliffs, N.J.: Prentice-Hall, Inc., 1965), p. 191.

Chapter 8

The Cost Finding Process

Cost finding is an integral part of the budgetary control system because it is the process by which the costs of nonrevenue-producing departments are allocated to each other and to revenue-producing departments. In fact, it is the only process that provides reasonable assurance that all direct and indirect costs are allocated to the appropriate revenue centers. As such, the cost finding process is the basis for rate setting.

Traditionally, the hospital industry has considered cost finding to be merely the process required to establish the amount to be reconciled at the end of the year between the hospital and third party payers such as Blue Cross and Medicare. Cost finding, however, is much more than that. It is a basic management tool that can help ensure the hospital's financial viability—if it is properly used.

A unique feature of cost finding is that it can be applied to both budgeted and historical costs. It is applied to budgeted costs for prospective rate setting, which is the establishment of rates before service is rendered. The most common use of prospective rate setting is to establish a "published" charge list, that is, the charges that appear on a patient's bill. Recently, there has been increased use of prospective rate setting by state hospital commissions and Blue Cross plans. In most of these instances, the established rate is final with no retrospective settlement. If the hospital's costs exceed the prospective rate, the hospital must assume the loss. On the other hand, if the hospital's costs are less than the prospective rate, the hospital can keep the surplus.

Cost finding is applied to historical costs in hospitals primarily to determine the cost of providing services that are reimbursed under third party contracts. The resulting information is used to determine the third party's financial obligation to the hospital at the time of the final settlement for the fiscal year. In some cases, the results of the cost finding process lead to retrospective negotiations or settlements with a third party. For example, a third party may agree to reimburse a hospital for its costs or charges—whichever is less. If the hospital billed the third party for $3 million, received interim payments totaling $2.5 million, and subsequently determined that its actual cost of providing the services was $2.75 million, the retrospective settlement would amount to $250,000:

1. Total patient charges $3,000,000
2. Third party interim payments to hospital 2,500,000
3. Hospital's third party cost 2,750,000
4. Due from third party 250,000

To illustrate further the retrospective settlement process, assume the following:

1. Total patient charges $2,650,000
2. Third party interim payments 2,500,000
3. Hospital's third party cost 2,750,000
4. Due from third party 150,000

In the first example, the hospital's charges were greater than its costs; therefore, it received its costs ($2,750,000). The retrospective settlement of $250,000 represents the difference between the hospital's costs and the third party's interim payments. In the second example, the hospital's charges of $2,650,000 were less than its costs, so it was entitled to receive only its charges. The retrospective settlement of $150,000 is the difference between the hospital's charges and the third party's interim payments.

These examples highlight the need for hospitals to keep established charges sufficiently higher than costs to not only generate the profit necessary to protect their assets but also to preclude being required to accept less than their costs from third party payers. To guard against the penalty of less-than-cost reimbursement, the hospital must monitor costs and charges monthly. This task can be accomplished by applying the cost finding process to the hospital's actual costs and comparing the results with the hospital's third party charges and interim payments. This should be done every month.

The American Hospital Association has identified the following objectives of cost finding in hospitals:[1]

- to provide full cost information as a basis for establishing rates for services and for assessing the adequacy of existing rates
- to provide information for use in negotiating reimbursement contracts with contracting agencies and in determining the amount of reimbursable costs

- to provide information for reports to hospital associations, governmental agencies, and other external groups
- to provide information for use in managerial decision making in areas other than rate setting

METHODS OF COST FINDING

While this chapter will concentrate on the results of cost finding, it is important for the patient account manager to be familiar with the mechanics of cost finding, too. With this knowledge, he/she can more easily answer criticism about "ridiculously high" charges for patient services.

According to the American Hospital Association, there are three basic types of hospital cost finding.

Method 1. This system allocates the costs of the nonrevenue-producing centers only to the revenue-producing centers. While it is obvious that most nonrevenue-producing centers render services to each other as well as to revenue-producing centers, this system ignores that fact. None of the costs of the nonrevenue-producing centers are allocated to the other nonrevenue-producing centers.[2]

Method 2. This system, usually referred to as the stepdown or single apportionment method, recognizes the important fact that services rendered by certain nonrevenue-producing centers are used by other nonrevenue-producing centers, as well as by revenue-producing centers or departments. The accumulated costs in a nonrevenue-producing center, therefore, are allocated to those nonrevenue-producing centers and revenue-producing centers that use its services. The significant feature of this method is that once the costs of a nonrevenue-producing center have been allocated to other centers, the center is considered "closed." This means that no portion of the costs of other nonrevenue-producing centers whose costs have yet to be allocated will be applied to it.[3]

Method 3. This method, the most complex of the three original American Hospital Association methods, is frequently called the double distribution or double apportionment method. It gives more recognition to the fact that nonrevenue-producing centers render services to other nonrevenue-producing centers as well as to revenue-producing centers. Under this method, nonrevenue-producing centers are not considered permanently closed after their costs have been allocated. Instead, they are reopened in the second part of the apportionment process to receive allocated costs from other nonrevenue-producing centers from which they have received services. After the costs of each nonrevenue-producing center have been allocated once, some costs will remain in some departments, representing services received from other departments. It is necessary to make a second apportionment to close out every nonrevenue-producing center's total direct and accumulated costs.[4]

Other methods of cost finding are based on the use of algebraic formulas and the computer. These formulas are designed to identify costs in departments that serve each other by recognizing the relationship that exists between those departments. Through the use of simultaneous equations, the cost allocation process for the nonrevenue-producing departments continues to accumulate cost and allocate it to other nonrevenue-producing centers as well as to revenue-producing centers until there is virtually no more cost left to allocate. The simultaneous equation method is by far the most sophisticated method of cost finding.

A much simpler method of cost allocation is the "Short Formula 1" method, based on the hospital's most recent comprehensive cost finding report. With this method, percentages of a revenue-producing department's costs are established. These allocated indirect or overhead percentages are then applied to the hospital's current actual or budgeted total nonrevenue-producing department costs and added to the costs of the respective revenue-producing departments to produce a total cost. This method is relatively accurate and requires minimal time compared with comprehensive cost finding. It is especially useful when approximations are sufficient. However, if there is a major change in statistical or expense distribution, for example, increased square footage, the overhead percentage must be adjusted to reflect the change. The "Short Formula 1" method is a "quick and dirty" manual approach to cost finding and departmental profitability testing when precise accuracy is not a major requirement.[5]

KEYS TO THE COST FINDING PROCESS

One of the three keys to the validity of the results of any cost finding or rate setting process is the departmental sequence by which costs are allocated. As stated earlier, there is no generally accepted procedure for establishing the departmental cost allocation sequence. Usually, the system is designed to meet the needs of its designer.

The cost finding allocation process should be designed in the following manner. The *first* center to be closed should be the center that renders the greatest amount of service to the largest number of centers and receives the least amount of service from the smallest number of centers. The *last* center to be closed should be the center that renders the least amount of service to the smallest number of centers and receives the greatest amount of service from the largest number of centers.[6]

The second key to the validity of any cost finding and rate setting process is the quality of the statistics used to distribute the nonrevenue-producing departments' costs to the revenue-producing departments. The quality of the allocation and, in fact, the entire cost finding process depends on the quality of the statistics. In selecting statistical bases, it is important to use the statistics that are most appropriate for each particular hospital. Furthermore, the statistical bases selected for each department or cost center should be the ones that are most appropriate for that department or cost center. Each statistical basis should be the one that most accurately represents the proportionate amount of service rendered by a given nonrevenue-producing center to other nonrevenue-producing centers and to revenue-producing centers. It is also important that the chosen statistic be easily identified, gathered and counted, audited, and subject to minimal probability of error.

The third and last key to valid cost finding and rate setting is the selection of the proper production unit for each revenue-producing department. The production unit is a minor part of the cost finding process, but it plays a major role in the rate setting process. The distinction between macro and micro production units was discussed in Chapter 5. In the cost finding and rate setting process, micro production units, that is, relative value units such as person-minutes, usually serve as the basis for rate setting. In the cost finding process, direct and allocated or indirect costs are identified for each revenue center. For example:

Laboratory

Direct costs	$716,509
Allocated indirect	195,955
Total costs	$912,464

Assume that a volume of 8,850,000 relative value units has been projected for this laboratory for the budget year. The data provided above can be used to develop the average cost per production unit:

$$\frac{\text{Total departmental costs}}{\text{Total relevant departmental production units}} = \text{Average cost per production unit}$$

or

$$\frac{\$912{,}464}{8{,}850{,}000} = \$0.103$$

168   PATIENT ACCOUNT MANAGEMENT

Table 8–1 General Fund Expense Summary, Memorial Hospital, Anytown, U.S.A.

(OMIT CENTS)

GENERAL FUND EXPENSE SUMMARY 12 MONTHS ENDED SEPT. 30, 19X3	1 SALARY & FEE EXPENSE	2 NON-SALARY EXPENSE	3 DEPRECIATION EXPENSE (FORM 5)	4 DEBIT & (CREDIT) ADJUSTMENTS (FORM 8)	5 CREDITS TO EXPENSE (FORM 8)	6 NET EXPENSE
GENERAL SERVICE DEPARTMENTS						
1 *ADMINISTRATION & GENERAL	518,015	580,551	28,391	20,982	2,811	1,145,128
2 DIETARY	213,980	221,310	9,944		141	445,093
3 HOUSEKEEPING	150,733	29,466	1,905			182,104
4 LAUNDRY	80,957	8,984	6,571			96,512
4A LINEN SERVICE	9,258	12,956	1,634		4,770	19,078
5 MAINTENANCE OF PERSONNEL	9,312	723	12,188		3,046	19,177
6 OPERATION OF PLANT	37,601	64,084	13,929			115,614
7 REPAIRS & MAINTENANCE	158,411	79,509	4,391		13,456	228,875
PROFESSIONAL SERVICE DEPARTMENTS						
8 NURSING SERVICE ADMINISTRATION	101,111	5,023	2,093			108,227
9 NURSING EDUCATION						
10 INTERNS, RESIDENTS & PHYSICIANS	63,016	20,266	1,396	(11,274)		73,404
11 MEDICAL RECORDS & LIBRARY	91,018	16,460	4,810		8,449	103,839
12 SOCIAL SERVICE	16,307	132	405			16,844
SPECIAL SERVICE DEPARTMENTS						
13 OPERATING ROOMS	142,392	85,266	10,007			237,665
14 POST OPERATIVE ROOM	62,269	598	1,511			64,378
15 ANESTHESIOLOGY	146,430	19,872	957			167,259
15 DELIVERY ROOMS	64,418	13,339	4,394		368	81,783
17 RADIOLOGY	262,152	121,038	15,364	(16,310)	2,323	379,921
18 LABORATORY	463,361	123,035	16,988	(8,979)		504,405
19 ELECTROENCEPHALOGRAPHY	11,959	513	889			13,361
20 ELECTROCARDIOLOGY	67,244	6,013	1,392	645		75,294
21 PHYSICAL THERAPY	26,352	572	2,413	(52)		29,285
22 MEDICAL & SURGICAL SUPPLIES		35,009				35,009
23 CENTRAL STERILE SUPPLY	42,839	903	3,191			46,933
24 INHALATION THERAPY	31,576	16,561	2,908	1,311		52,356
25 INTRAVENOUS THERAPY	59,214	63,488	139			122,841
26 PHARMACY	38,335	145,642	1,561	(127)	173	185,238
27 EMERGENCY SERVICE	59,818	19,415	4,432	(6)		83,659
28 ISOTOPE THERAPY	39,599	46,806	3,881			90,286
29 COST OF DRUGS SOLD						
30 ROUTINE SPECIAL SERVICES						
31 M-HEALTH	46,492	562	1,022		55,000	(6,924)
32 R. THERAPY	5,496	3,987	108			9,591
33						
34						
35 RADIUM THERAPY						
36 SHOCK THERAPY						
37 OCCUPATIONAL THERAPY						
38 NON-CBC SPECIAL SERVICES						
39						
40						
41						
42						
43						
ROUTINE SERVICE						
44 NON-MATERNITY	964,138	82,202	51,289	(1,966)		1,095,663
45						
46						
47						
48						
TOTAL (Lines 44-48)						
49 MATERNITY	61,523	8,762	4,375			74,660
50 NEWBORN INFANTS	55,819	9,625	1,588			67,032
51 OUTPATIENT CLINICS	12,013	2,771	1,871			16,655
52 PRIVATE REFERRED OUTPATIENTS						
OTHER EXPENSE						
53 REAL ESTATE & PROPERTY TAXES						
54 RESEARCH						
55 FUND RAISING EXPENSE			638			638
56 AMBULANCE SERVICE						
57 SPECIAL NURSES & GUEST MEALS						
58 PAY CAFETERIA	33,499	1,761	4,188	15,776	85,706	(30,482)
59 COFFEE & GIFT SHOPS			1,375			1,375
60 BLOOD & BLOOD DERIVATIVES						
61						
62						
63 MISCELLANEOUS						
64 TOTAL	4,146,677	1,847,204	224,138	-0-	176,243	6,041,776

*INTEREST EXPENSE IN THE AMOUNT OF $ 35,881 INCLUDED.

POST TO FORM 9 COL 1

After computing average cost per micro production unit, it is relatively simple to continue the process and establish an average charge or selling price for the production unit. This procedure is discussed in more detail in Chapter 9.

A COST FINDING CASE STUDY

The cost finding case study presented here uses Method 3, the double apportionment method of cost finding. As with any other cost finding system, the process illustrated in the case study starts with the gathering of the hospital's direct departmental costs as illustrated in Table 8–1. In the case study, the total net expenses are $6,041,776 (see column 6, line 64). (This amount will serve as a "proof total" at each cost allocation checkpoint in Table 8–3, column 12, line 64 and in Table 8–4, column 15, line 64.)

An interesting feature of the case study is its distribution of depreciation (see Table 8–2). Note that major or movable and fixed equipment expenses are allocated directly to the using department; however, depreciation expense for buildings is allocated on the basis of square feet. The total depreciation expense of $224,138 is distributed to individual centers as shown in Table 8–1, column 3, lines 1 through 64.

The statistical bases listed below were used to allocate the remaining cost centers:

Cost Center	Statistical Base
Administration	Average number of employees (full-time equivalents)
Housekeeping	Hours of service
Laundry and linen	Pounds of clean laundry processed
Operation of plant	Square feet
Repairs and maintenance	Square feet
Dietary	Number of meals served
Loss on pay cafeteria	Number of meals served
Maintenance of personnel	Number of personnel living in
Nursing service administration	Hours of service
Nursing education	Weighted student hours
Interns and residents	Hours of service
Pharmacy	Requisitioned costs
Central sterile supply	Requisitioned costs
Medical records and library	Weighted discharges
Social service	Weighted visits
Administration (second allocation)	Accumulated costs

170   PATIENT ACCOUNT MANAGEMENT

Table 8–2 Schedule of Depreciation, Memorial Hospital, Anytown, U.S.A.

(OMIT CENTS)

SCHEDULE OF DEPRECIATION 12 MONTHS ENDED SEPT. 30, 198__	1 MOVABLE EQUIPMENT	2 FIXED EQUIPMENT	3 *BUILDINGS	4 TOTAL
GENERAL SERVICE DEPARTMENTS				
1 ADMINISTRATION & GENERAL	7,900	813	19,678	28,391
2 DIETARY	4,612	420	4,912	9,944
3 HOUSEKEEPING	1,075	5	825	1,905
4 LAUNDRY	4,429	140	2,002	6,571
4A LINEN SERVICE			1,634	1,634
5 MAINTENANCE OF PERSONNEL	689	5	11,494	12,188
6 OPERATION OF PLANT	285	9,664	3,980	13,929
7 REPAIRS & MAINTENANCE	1,125	217	3,049	4,391
PROFESSIONAL SERVICE DEPARTMENTS				
8 NURSING SERVICE ADMINISTRATION	468		1,625	2,093
9 NURSING EDUCATION				
10 INTERNS, RESIDENTS & PHYSICIANS	131		1,265	1,396
11 MEDICAL RECORDS & LIBRARY	1,506	75	3,229	4,810
12 SOCIAL SERVICE	12		393	405
SPECIAL SERVICE DEPARTMENTS				
13 OPERATING ROOMS	3,908	2,265	3,834	10,007
14 POST OPERATIVE ROOM	357	194	960	1,511
15 ANESTHESIOLOGY	648		309	957
16 DELIVERY ROOMS	1,204	512	2,678	4,394
17 RADIOLOGY	10,069	1,142	4,153	15,364
18 LABORATORY	8,345	1,969	6,674	16,988
19 ELECTROENCEPHALOGRAPHY	565		324	889
20 ELECTROCARDIOLOGY	1,068		324	1,392
21 PHYSICAL THERAPY	553	194	1,666	2,413
22 MEDICAL & SURGICAL SUPPLIES				
23 CENTRAL STERILE SUPPLY	977	285	1,929	3,191
24 INHALATION THERAPY	2,237		671	2,908
25 INTRAVENOUS THERAPY			139	139
26 PHARMACY	258	242	1,061	1,561
27 EMERGENCY SERVICE	722	1,554	2,156	4,432
28 ISOTOPE THERAPY	3,326		555	3,881
29 COST OF DRUGS SOLD				
30 ROUTINE SPECIAL SERVICES				
31 MENTAL HEALTH	69	141	812	1,022
32 RAD. THERAPY			108	108
33				
34				
35 RADIUM THERAPY				
36 SHOCK THERAPY				
37 OCCUPATIONAL THERAPY				
38 NON-CSC SPECIAL SERVICES				
39				
40				
41				
42				
43				
ROUTINE SERVICE				
44 NON-MATERNITY	9,647	4,978	36,664	51,289
45				
46				
47				
48				
TOTAL (Lines 44-48)				
49 MATERNITY	901	229	3,245	4,375
50 NEWBORN INFANTS	299	106	1,183	1,588
51 OUTPATIENT CLINICS	168	7	1,696	1,871
52 PRIVATE REFERRED OUTPATIENTS				
OTHER EXPENSE				
53 REAL ESTATE & PROPERTY TAXES				
54 RESEARCH				
55 FUND RAISING EXPENSE	46		592	638
56 AMBULANCE SERVICE				
57 SPECIAL NURSES & GUEST MEALS				
58 PAY CAFETERIA	1,378		2,810	4,188
59 COFFEE & GIFT SHOPS	832		543	1,375
60 BLOOD & BLOOD DERIVATIVES				
61				
62				
63 MISCELLANEOUS				
64 TOTAL	69,809	25,157	129,172	224,138

POST TO FORM 3 COL 3

Depreciation of Fixed Equipment and Buildings should be on the basis of Floor Area as defined on Page 13 of the Cost Analysis Manual. The depreciation on buildings occupied solely by one department should be charged in full to that department.

*Includes Depreciation on Land Improvements in the amount of $ 26,834

Since most hospitals are not organized or operated the same way, many costs may not be equitably or appropriately distributed in a specific hospital if typical statistical bases are used. If this is the case, alternate statistical bases may permit more equitable allocation of costs. Where third party reimbursement is concerned, changing the bases for allocating costs requires intermediary approval before the beginning of the reporting period to which the change applies. However, ongoing studies should be examined to refine and improve the cost finding process. These studies should be adequately documented and should support the hospital's decision to change the basis of allocation. Because the decision to change the statistical basis for allocating a cost or the order in which costs are allocated must be made before the beginning of the reporting period to which the change applies, it is absolutely necessary to carefully analyze the full effect of the change before requesting it. A computer program can be used for this analysis as well as for determining the impact of reclassification entries.

There is no single generally accepted cost finding procedure. The Medicare approach to cost finding is probably the most commonly used method; unfortunately, as is the case with other third party reimbursement cost finding methods, it is designed to minimize reimbursement to the hospital rather than to develop the true cost of a revenue-producing hospital department. For this reason, the Medicare cost finding system should *not* be used for rate setting. As noted earlier, the cost finding method illustrated in the case study presented in this chapter differs from the Medicare method.

To continue with the case study, examine Table 8–3, which illustrates the first apportionment of costs. It should be noted that the nonrevenue-producing cost centers are *not* closed out after the first apportionment as in the stepdown method. Instead, they are kept open for a second or double apportionment as shown in Table 8–4. In the double apportionment method, the nonrevenue-producing departments pick up the costs of other nonrevenue-producing departments as well as those of revenue-producing departments. For example, Table 8–3 (column 1, line 3) indicates that housekeeping has total direct expenses of $182,104 and accumulates the following indirect expenses:

Administration	$69,933
Laundry and linen	466
Operation of plant	792
Repairs and maintenance	1,560
Loss on pay cafeteria	9,089
Total	$81,842

Housekeeping's total accumulated indirect or allocated expenses of $81,842 are transferred to Table 8–4 (column 2, line 64) for the second apportion-

172 PATIENT ACCOUNT MANAGEMENT

Table 8-3 Preliminary Apportionment,

PRELIMINARY APPORTIONMENT 12 MONTHS ENDED SEPT. 30, 198__	1 NET EXPENSE	2 ADMINIS-TRATION	3 HOUSE-KEEPING	4 LAUNDRY & LINEN SERVICE	5 OPERATION OF PLANT	6 REPAIRS & MAINTENANCE SERVICE
		WORK SHEET 1	WORK SHEET 2	WORK SHEET 3	WORK SHEET 4	WORK SHEET 5
GENERAL SERVICE DEPARTMENTS						
1 ADMINISTRATION & GENERAL	1,145,128		29,057		18,931	37,190
2 DIETARY	445,093	96,825	7,253	522	4,726	9,283
3 HOUSEKEEPING	182,104	69,933		466	794	1,560
4 LAUNDRY & LINEN SERVICE	115,590	38,303	5,369		3,498	6,871
5 MAINTENANCE OF PERSONNEL	19,177	4,481	9,554	1,138	6,225	12,228
6 OPERATION OF PLANT	115,614	10,696	5,877	129		7,522
7 REPAIRS & MAINTENANCE	228,875	44,223	4,502	142	2,933	
PROFESSIONAL SERVICE DEPARTMENTS						
8 NURSING SERVICE ADMINISTRATION	108,227	27,331	2,399	49	1,563	3,071
9 NURSING EDUCATION						
10 INTERNS, RESIDENTS & PHYSICIANS	73,404	16,906	1,868	288	1,217	2,391
11 MEDICAL RECORDS & LIBRARY	103,839	39,094	4,768		3,107	6,103
12 SOCIAL SERVICE	16,844	5,241	581	46	379	744
SPECIAL SERVICE DEPARTMENTS						
13 OPERATING ROOMS	237,665					
14 POST OPERATIVE ROOM	64,378	12,753	1,418	741	924	1,815
15 ANESTHESIOLOGY	167,259	18,571	456	236	297	583
16 DELIVERY ROOMS	81,783	18,551	3,955	4,919	2,577	5,052
17 RADIOLOGY	379,921	52,243	6,132	1,641	3,955	7,848
18 LABORATORY	594,405	117,816	9,856	329	6,421	12,615
19 ELECTROENCEPHALOGRAPHY	13,361	3,981	478	175	312	612
20 ELECTROCARDIOLOGY	75,294	13,774	478	171	312	612
21 PHYSICAL THERAPY	29,285	9,448	2,461	526	1,603	3,149
22 MEDICAL & SURGICAL SUPPLIES	35,009					
23 CENTRAL STERILE SUPPLY	46,933	18,592	2,849	296	1,856	3,646
24 INHALATION THERAPY	52,356	11,930	991	184	646	1,268
25 INTRAVENOUS THERAPY	122,841	16,907	205		134	262
26 PHARMACY	185,238	12,139	1,566	56	1,021	2,005
27 EMERGENCY SERVICE	83,659	19,290	3,184	2,754	2,074	4,075
28 ISOTOPE THERAPY	90,286	8,501	820		534	1,050
29 COST OF DRUGS SOLD						
30 ROUTINE SPECIAL SERVICES						
31 Mental Health	(6,924)	8,150	1,199		782	1,535
32 Radiation Therapy	9,591	1,955	159		104	204
33						
34						
35 RADIUM THERAPY						
36 SHOCK THERAPY						
37 OCCUPATIONAL THERAPY						
38 NON-CHG SPECIAL SERVICES						
39						
40						
41						
42						
43						
ROUTINE SERVICE						
44 OBS-MATERNITY	1,095,663	335,106	54,138	71,984	35,273	69,292
45						
46						
47						
48						
TOTAL (Lines 44-48)						
49 MATERNITY	74,660	19,299	4,792	3,274	3,122	6,134
50 NEWBORN INFANTS	67,032	18,825	1,747	2,248	1,139	2,237
51 OUTPATIENT CLINICS	16,655	3,899	2,505	391	1,631	3,206
52 PRIVATE REFERRED OUTPATIENTS						
OTHER EXPENSE						
53 REAL ESTATE & PROPERTY TAXES						
54 RESEARCH						
55 FUND RAISING EXPENSE	638		875		570	1,120
56 AMBULANCE SERVICE						
57 SPECIAL NURSES & GUEST MEALS						
58 PAY CAFETERIA	(30,482)	17,542	4,149	105	2,703	5,310
59 COFFEE & GIFT SHOPS	1,375		802	101	522	1,026
60 BLOOD & BLOOD DERIVATIVES						
61						
62						
63 MISCELLANEOUS						
64 TOTAL	6,041,776	1,145,128	182,104	115,590	115,614	228,875
	NET EXPENSE FROM FORM 3, COL. 6	TOTAL EQUALS COL. 1, LINE 1	TOTAL EQUALS COL. 1, LINE 3	TOTAL EQUALS COL. 1, LINE 4	TOTAL EQUALS COL. 1, LINE 6	TOTAL EQUALS COL. 1, LINE 7

The Cost Finding Process

Memorial Hospital, Anytown, U.S.A.

(OMIT CENTS)

7 TOTAL COLUMNS 2-6	8 DIETARY	9 LOSS ON PAY CAFETERIA	10 MAINTENANCE OF PERSONNEL	11 COLUMN 1 LINES 8 TO 64	12 TOTAL COLUMNS 7 TO 11		
	WORK SHEET 6	WORK SHEET 7	WORK SHEET 8			GENERAL SERVICE DEPARTMENTS	
85,178					108,431	ADMINISTRATION & GENERAL	1
118,609						DIETARY	2
72,753		9,089			81,842	HOUSEKEEPING	3
54,041		4,934			58,975	LAUNDRY & LINEN SERVICE	4
33,626		584				MAINTENANCE OF PERSONNEL	5
24,224		1,307			25,531	OPERATION OF PLANT	6
51,800		5,384			57,184	REPAIRS & MAINTENANCE	7
						PROFESSIONAL SERVICE DEPARTMENTS	
34,413		3,309		108,227	145,949	NURSING SERVICE ADMINISTRATION	8
						NURSING EDUCATION	9
22,670	19,810	2,149	15,951	73,404	133,984	INTERNS, RESIDENTS & PHYSICIANS	10
53,072		5,042		103,839	161,953	MEDICAL RECORDS & LIBRARY	11
6,991		652		16,844	24,487	SOCIAL SERVICE	12
92,098				237,665	342,650	SPECIAL SERVICE DEPARTMENTS OPERATING ROOMS	13
17,651		1,457		64,378	83,486	POST OPERATIVE ROOM	14
20,143	1,534	2,273	5,860	167,259	197,069	ANESTHESIOLOGY	15
35,064		2,271		81,783	119,118	DELIVERY ROOMS	16
71,859	5,920	6,527	3,906	379,921	468,133	RADIOLOGY	17
147,037	1,991	14,857	11,719	594,405	770,009	LABORATORY	18
5,558		498		13,361	19,417	ELECTROENCEPHALOGRAPHY	19
15,347		1,603	1,953	75,294	94,197	ELECTROCARDIOLOGY	20
17,187		1,194	1,953	29,285	49,619	PHYSICAL THERAPY	21
				35,009	35,009	MEDICAL & SURGICAL SUPPLIES	22
27,239		2,401		46,933	76,573	CENTRAL STERILE SUPPLY	23
15,019		1,517	1,953	52,356	70,845	INHALATION THERAPY	24
17,508		2,056		122,841	142,415	INTRAVENOUS THERAPY	25
16,787		1,508		185,238	203,533	PHARMACY	26
31,377		2,402	1,953	83,654	119,391	EMERGENCY SERVICE	27
10,905		982		90,286	102,173	ISOTOPE THERAPY	28
						COST OF DRUGS SOLD	29
						ROUTINE SPECIAL SERVICES	30
11,666		1,001		(6,924)	5,743		31
2,422		247		9,591	12,260		32
							33
							34
						RADIUM THERAPY	35
						SHOCK THERAPY	36
						OCCUPATIONAL THERAPY	37
						NON-CBC SPECIAL SERVICES	38
							39
							40
							41
							42
							43
565,793	355,317	42,162		1,095,663	2,058,935	ROUTINE SERVICE NON-MATERNITY	44
							45
							46
							47
							48
						TOTAL (Lines 44-48)	
36,621	25,848	2,394	1,953	74,660	141,476	MATERNITY	49
26,196		2,359		67,032	95,587	NEWBORN INFANTS	50
11,632		486		16,655	28,773	OUTPATIENT CLINICS	51
						PRIVATE REFERRED OUTPATIENTS	52
						OTHER EXPENSE REAL ESTATE & PROPERTY TAXES	53
						RESEARCH	54
2,565				638	3,203	FUND RAISING EXPENSE	55
						AMBULANCE SERVICE	56
						SPECIAL NURSES & GUEST MEALS	57
29,809	153,282					PAY CAFETERIA	58
2,451				1,375	3,826	COFFEE & GIFT SHOPS	59
						BLOOD & BLOOD DERIVATIVES	60
							61
							62
						MISCELLANEOUS	63
6,787,311	563,702	152,609	53,387	3,820,677	6,041,776	TOTAL	64
TOTAL EQUALS COLS. 2-6 LINE 64	TOTAL EQUALS COLS. 147 LINE 2	TOTAL EQUALS COLS. 1,7, & 8 LINE 58	TOTAL EQUALS COLS. 1,7,8,&9 LINE 5		TOTAL EQUALS COL. 1, LINE 64		

174 PATIENT ACCOUNT MANAGEMENT

Table 8-4 Secondary Apportionment,

	1 FORM 9 LINES 13-64 IN COL. 12	2 HOUSE- KEEPING	3 LAUNDRY & LINEN SERVICE	4 OPERATION OF PLANT	5 REPAIRS & MAINTENANCE SERVICE	6 NURSING SERVICE ADMINISTRATION	7 NURSING EDUCATION	8 INTERNS RESIDENTS & PHYSICIANS
		WORK SHEET 9	WORK SHEET 10	WORK SHEET 11	WORK SHEET 12	WORK SHEET 13	WORK SHEET 14	WORK SHEET 15
13	342,650							
14	83,486	1,088	387	339	760			
15	197,059	349	123	109	244			
16	119,118	3,033	2,574	946	2,119	5,477		6,959
17	468,133	4,702	859	1,467	3,285			
18	770,009	7,558	172	2,359	5,282			43,133
19	19,417	367	91	114	256			
20	94,197	367	89	114	256			15,191
21	49,619	1,887	275	589	1,318			
22	35,009							
23	76,573	2,185	155	682	1,526	5,759		
24	70,845	760	97	237	531			
25	142,415	157		49	110	4,957		10,135
26	203,533	1,201	29	375	839			
27	119,391	2,441	1,442	762	1,705			2,347
28	102,173	629		196	439			1,269
29								
30								
31	5,743	920		287	643			
32	12,260	122		38	85			
33								
44	2,058,935	41,514	37,668	12,951	29,006	101,143		17,530
49	141,476	3,675	1,713	1,146	2,568	5,742		2,603
50	95,587	1,340	1,176	417	936	5,659		3,446
51	28,773	1,920	204	599	1,342	1,166		11,138
55	3,203	671		209	469			
59	3,826	615	53	192	430			
64	5,243,440	81,842	58,975	25,531	57,184	145,949	None	133,984
		TOTAL EQUALS FORM 9 COLUMN 12 LINE 3	TOTAL EQUALS FORM 9 COLUMN 12 LINE 4	TOTAL EQUALS FORM 9 COLUMN 12 LINE 6	TOTAL EQUALS FORM 9 COLUMN 12 LINE 7	TOTAL EQUALS FORM 9 COLUMN 12 LINE 8	TOTAL EQUALS FORM 9 COLUMN 12 LINE 9	TOTAL EQUALS FORM 9 COLUMN 12 LINE 10

NOTE A: Add Line 26, Columns 1-8 and post as a credit on Line 26, Column 9. Redistribute on Worksheet 16.

NOTE B: Add Line 23, Columns 1-9 and post as a credit on Line 23, Column 10. Redistribute on Worksheet 17.

Memorial Hospital, Anytown, U.S.A.

(OMIT CENTS)

SECONDARY APPORTIONMENT 12 MONTHS ENDED SEPT. 30, 1968	9 PHARMACY	10 CENTRAL STERILE SUPPLY	11 MEDICAL RECORDS & LIBRARY	12 SOCIAL SERVICE	13 TOTAL COLUMNS 1 TO 12	14 ADMINISTRATION	15 TOTAL COLUMNS 13 AND 14	
	WORK SHEET 16	WORK SHEET 17	WORK SHEET 18	WORK SHEET 19		WORK SHEET 20		
SPECIAL SERVICE DEPARTMENTS					435,163		443,116	12
OPERATING ROOMS					87,030	1,590	88,620	14
POST OPERATIVE ROOM	97	873			201,338	3,679	205,017	15
ANESTHESIOLOGY	3,444				152,288	2,783	155,071	16
DELIVERY ROOMS	2,037	10,043			491,932	8,990	500,922	17
RADIOLOGY	386	13,100			830,124	15,170	845,294	18
LABORATORY	738	873			20,271	370	20,641	19
ELECTROENCEPHALOGRAPHY	26				112,392	2,054	114,446	20
ELECTROCARDIOLOGY	2	437	1,739		53,712	982	54,694	21
PHYSICAL THERAPY	24				58,589	1,071	59,660	22
MEDICAL & SURGICAL SUPPLIES		23,580						23
CENTRAL STERILE SUPPLY	453	(87,333)			72,917	1,333	74,250	24
INHALATION THERAPY	447				157,964	2,887	160,851	25
INTRAVENOUS THERAPY	141							26
PHARMACY	(205,977)				144,028	2,632	146,660	27
EMERGENCY SERVICE	9,887	2,620	3,432		104,712	1,914	105,626	28
ISOTOPE THERAPY	6							29
COST OF DRUGS SOLD	172,034				172,034	3,144	175,178	30
ROUTINE SPECIAL SERVICES					7,593	139	7,732	31
Mental Health					12,505	229	12,734	32
Radiation Therapy								33
								34
RADIUM THERAPY								35
SHOCK THERAPY								36
OCCUPATIONAL THERAPY								37
NON-CBC SPECIAL SERVICES								38
								39
								40
								41
								42
								43
ROUTINE SERVICE								
NON-MATERNITY	8,084		142,327	20,066	2,469,224	45,125	2,514,349	44
								45
								46
								47
								48
TOTAL (Lines 44-48)					167,662	3,064	170,726	
MATERNITY	2,410		4,938	1,391	117,165	2,140	119,305	49
NEWBORN INFANTS	936	3,493	4,140	35	51,373	939	52,312	50
OUTPATIENT CLINICS	647	873	1,716	2,995	3,661	67	3,728	51
PRIVATE REFERRED OUTPATIENTS			3,661					52
OTHER EXPENSE								53
REAL ESTATE & PROPERTY TAXES								54
RESEARCH					4,552	83	4,635	55
FUND RAISING EXPENSE								56
AMBULANCE SERVICE								57
SPECIAL NURSES & GUEST MEALS								58
PAY CAFETERIA								59
COFFEE & GIFT SHOPS					5,116	93	5,209	60
BLOOD & BLOOD DERIVATIVES								61
								62
MISCELLANEOUS								63
TOTAL	-0-	-0-	161,953	24,487	5,933,345	108,431	6,041,776	64
	TOTAL EQUALS ZERO (NOTE A)	TOTAL EQUALS ZERO (NOTE B)	TOTAL EQUALS FORM 9 COLUMN 12 LINE 11	TOTAL EQUALS FORM 9 COLUMN 12 LINE 12		TOTAL EQUALS FORM 9 COLUMN 12 LINE 1	TOTAL EQUALS FORM 3 COLUMN 6 LINE 64	

ment to departments that use housekeeping's services. The first and second apportionment of nonrevenue-producing costs to using departments is concluded in Table 8–4 (column 10, lines 13 and 14). Table 8–5 summarizes the hospital's revenue-producing departments' direct and indirect expenses. Note that one of the checkpoints or "proof totals" mentioned earlier is the $6,041,776, which appears at the end of Table 8–5.

As stated earlier, Medicare prescribes the use of the stepdown method of cost finding even though more sophisticated methods may be used. It must be noted here that intermediary approval is required before a hospital

Table 8–5 Summary of Revenue-Producing Departments' Direct and Indirect Expenses

Memorial Hospital, Anytown, U.S.A.
Summary of Revenue-Producing Departments' Direct and Indirect Expenses
For the Year Ending September 30, 19x1

Department	Direct Expense	Indirect Expense	Total Expense
Operating Rooms	$ 237,665	$ 205,451	$ 443,116
Postoperative Room	64,378	24,242	88,620
Anesthesiology	167,259	37,758	205,017
Delivery Room	81,783	73,288	155,071
Radiology	379,921	121,001	500,922
Laboratory	594,405	340,889	845,294
E.E.G.	13,361	7,280	20,641
E.K.G.	75,294	39,152	114,446
Physical Therapy	29,285	25,409	54,694
Central Sterile Supply	81,942	(22,282)	59,660
Inhalation Therapy	52,356	21,894	74,250
Intravenous Therapy	122,841	38,010	160,851
Pharmacy	185,238	(10,060)	175,178
Emergency Service	83,659	63,001	146,660
Isotope Therapy	90,286	16,340	106,626
Mental Health	(6,924)	14,656	7,732
Radiation Therapy	9,591	3,143	12,734
Nonmaternity Nursery	1,095,663	1,418,686	2,514,349
Maternity Nursery	74,660	96,066	170,726
Newborn Nursery	67,032	52,273	119,305
Outpatient Clinic	16,655	39,385	56,040
Total	$3,426,350	$2,605,582	$6,031,932
Plus:			
Other Expenses			
Fund Raising			4,635
Coffee and Gift Shop			5,209
Total Expenses			$6,041,776

can substitute another method of cost finding, such as the double apportionment method, for Medicare. It should also be noted that once a hospital has received intermediary approval to use a more sophisticated cost finding method, it may not return to a less sophisticated method, that is, stepdown cost finding. Therefore, the hospital is advised to test any cost finding methods it is considering to find the one that is most beneficial to the hospital before requesting any change in methodology; once a change is requested, there is no return.

Regardless of which system the hospital selects for cost finding, it is important to keep in mind the purposes the cost finding method is intended to achieve. If cost finding is to be used for rate setting, the system should be designed so that the costs of nonrevenue-producing departments are allocated in such a manner that they are accurately reflected in the hospital's published charges.

If, on the other hand, the cost finding process is the basis for third party reimbursement, the hospital will find that it must use designated forms and conform to regulatory reporting requirements. However, this does not preclude the use of imaginative or creative cost finding that maximizes reimbursement. The hospital is advised to document all deviations from prescribed reporting requirements and be prepared to support its position all the way through an appeal to the Provider Reimbursement Review Board (PRRB), the body which adjudicates Medicare reimbursement disputes.

In summary, the cost finding process is a management tool that can be used to the hospital's advantage or disadvantage. It all depends on who designs the cost finding methodology and what the designer intends to accomplish with it.

NOTES

1. *Cost Finding and Rate Setting for Hospitals* (Chicago: American Hospital Association, 1968), p. 2.
2. Ibid., p. 21.
3. Allen G. Herkimer, Jr., *Understanding Hospital Financial Management* (Germantown, Md.: Aspen Systems Corp., 1978), p. 166.
4. Ibid., pp. 167–168.
5. Ibid., pp. 169–171.
6. American Hospital Association, *Cost Finding and Rate Setting for Hospitals*, p. 22.

Chapter 9

Financial Requirements and Rate Setting

One of the main purposes of any business is to render service or to manufacture a commodity for a customer—to meet a consumer's need. Ideally, a fair exchange is negotiated, and the customer and the business are mutually satisfied.

The primary responsibility of any business executive is to develop and maintain the business's financial viability and growth. This can be accomplished by assuring that the business's long-range financial plan identifies and incorporates its financial requirements, as well as its operating costs, in its rate setting or pricing structure.

A hospital is a business. It must be conducted as a business if it is to survive and serve its patients, employees, and community responsibly. This means that the hospital must be paid its financial or economic requirements, as well as its accounting or operating costs. The one thing that accounting and economic requirements have in common is that they both recognize normal, day-to-day out-of-pocket costs such as:

- salaries and wages
- nonsalary supplies and expenses
- purchased services
- depreciation (amortized at cost)

Although these are generally accepted hospital accounting costs, the Medicare and Medicaid reimbursement systems take considerable objection to the acceptability of these costs. Moreover, most of the third party purchasers of hospital services do not completely accept the hospital's economic costs.

FINANCIAL REQUIREMENTS

The American Hospital Association (AHA), in its publication *Factors to Evaluate in the Establishment of Hospital Charges*, states:[1]

> ... the rates charged for each individual service should reflect properly the operating expenses of the service rendered, plus an equitable share of the other financial needs for which the patient is responsible.

As Berman and Weeks point out, this AHA statement is a reasonable and financially realistic philosophical guideline for establishing charges. However, it does not indicate the specific cost elements that must be considered if charges are to properly reflect operating expenses and other financial needs.[2] They also observe that (1) third party cost-based reimbursement systems would have to be substantially modified to cover all the economic costs of hospital operation so that reimbursement would equal full economic cost, and (2) hospital rates should be based on economic cost rather than financial expediency.[3]

According to Seawell, hospital economic costs include:[4]

- basic production costs of providing hospital services
- education
- research
- community health program expenses
- working and plant capital needs
- bad debts and free services

One economic cost that Seawell does not include is profit. To Drucker, profit is not merely an objective of a business, it is a requirement. Profit, he observes, is the *result* of doing things right rather than the purpose of business activity.[5] Profitability measures how well the hospital conducts its operations to serve the community and the patient. Above all, profit is a restraint. Unless the hospital can generate enough profit to cover its risks, demand for new technology, inflation expense, and maintenance or replacement of assets, it will not be able to attain its objectives.

Drucker calls profit the "cost of staying in business," that is, an actual, albeit deferred, cost.[6] A business that does not earn enough to cover this cost is bound to disappear eventually, or perhaps to be taken over by the government, as has happened in England and other countries where the ownership of hospitals has been assumed by the government. Drucker adds that it is often said that profit is a reward for the investor, in other words, a return on money invested in the past. However, according to Drucker, nothing could be further from the truth. What is mistakenly called profit is the genuine cost of the future of the enterprise and the economy. A rate of profit that does not equal the cost of capital is not profit at all. It is really loss, both for a hospital and for the economy.[7]

Drucker concludes that "not-for-profit" institutions, including hospitals, must consider the cost of staying in business as part of their operating costs.[8] Traditionally, hospitals have treated any surplus of operating revenues over operating expenses as something to apologize for. The true nature of these surpluses as costs has been obscured, a policy that has endangered the future of the nation's hospitals. The danger inherent in not treating profit as a cost of staying in business or a cost of the future rather than of current operations in public service institutions is dramatically illustrated by the failure of the British National Health Service to take into account, from 1950 until today, the known costs of necessary hospital construction.[9]

The plain fact is that any hospital—or any business, for that matter—requires payment not only for its operating costs but also for its economic costs if it is to grow, especially in an inflationary economy. Furthermore, the economic costs must be based on the budget, not experience. The present inequitable and discriminatory hospital payment system must be corrected or we will see the demise of the pluralistic hospital system in this country. If the payment system is not improved, total government ownership of hospitals will result—a disaster for America's superb health care delivery system.

THIRD PARTY IMPACT ON PUBLISHED RATES

Many major third party purchasers of hospital services, such as Medicare, Medicaid, and some Blue Cross plans, purchase these services under a contract. In effect, these contracts require a hospital to accept as full payment (except for patient deductibles and coinsurance) the amount the third party considers reasonable or appropriate. The difference between the full charge to a patient and the third party's payment for that patient's care is called a contractual allowance, as illustrated below:

	Accounting System	*Cash System*
Total gross charges to patient	$5,000	
Less: deductible and coinsurance due from patient	500	$ 500
Net charge to third party	4,500	

	Accounting System	Cash System
Due from third party based on cost settlement	$4,050	$4,050
Contractual allowance	$ 450	
Total cash inflow		$4,550

This process is remarkable in that:

- The third party is the major purchaser of these services.
- The third party determines what costs are "reasonable, appropriate, and allowable."
- Any difference between the third party's cash payment and the hospital's published charge (the contractual allowance) is lost income.
- The hospital has no *recourse* to the patient or any other party; its only course of action is to recover the contractual allowance somehow from the full-charge patient.

What is really happening? The private or self-pay patient and the patient with commercial insurance coverage are actually subsidizing the third party patients and their guarantors This fact is demonstrated by the following case study.

CASE STUDY OF REIMBURSEMENT PROCEDURES

Assume that Memorial Hospital of Anytown, U.S.A. has computed its actual accounting costs for 1,000 patient days as follows:

Total operating costs for 1,000 patient days

Salaries and Wages	$210,000
Nonsalary Expenses	80,000
Depreciation	10,000
Total Operating Costs	$300,000

Assume further that the hospital has been experiencing a loss of ten percent of operating total costs due to bad debts and charity allowances. In addition, the hospital's board of trustees has decided that the hospital requires a minimum of ten percent of total operating costs as profit to provide for growth and development. The hospital's total financial requirements may be summarized as follows:

Total Financial Requirements

Operating Costs	Total Amount	Average Cost Per Patient Day	Percent
Salaries and Wages	$210,000	$210	58.34%
Nonsalary Expenses	80,000	80	22.22
Depreciation	10,000	10	2.78
Total Operating Costs	$300,000	$300	83.34%
Plus: (a) Provision for Bad Debts and Charity Allowance	30,000	30	8.33
(b) Growth and Development	30,000	30	8.33
Total Financial Requirements	$360,000	$360	100.00%

These amounts are illustrated in Figure 9–1. This illustration assumes that all patients are charged the same average rate of $360 per patient day—a two party payment system.

To continue with the case study, assume that half of Memorial Hospital's patients are covered by a third party payment system. These third party payment systems reimburse the hospital only for its accounting costs of $300 per patient day, even though the hospital must provide for bad debts and charity care, as well as for its profit or growth and development—costs that are spread over the entire patient population. The following computation shows the redistribution of the hospital's financial requirements:

Description	Full-Charge Patient	Cost-Pay Patient	Total
Number of Patients	500	500	1,000
Direct Cost			
Salaries and Wages	$105,000	$105,000	$210,000
Nonsalary Expenses	40,000	40,000	80,000
Depreciation	5,000	5,000	10,000
Total Direct Cost	$150,000	$150,000	$300,000
Plus:			
(a) Provision for Bad Debts and Charity	30,000	None	30,000
(b) Profit	30,000	None	30,000

184 PATIENT ACCOUNT MANAGEMENT

Description	Full-Charge Patient	Cost-Pay Patient	Total
Total Financial Requirements	$210,000	$150,000	$360,000
Average per Patient Day	$ 420	$ 300	$ 360

Figure 9–1 Hospital's Financial Requirements per Patient Day for 1000 Patients—Two Party Payment System, Memorial Hospital, Anytown, U.S.A.

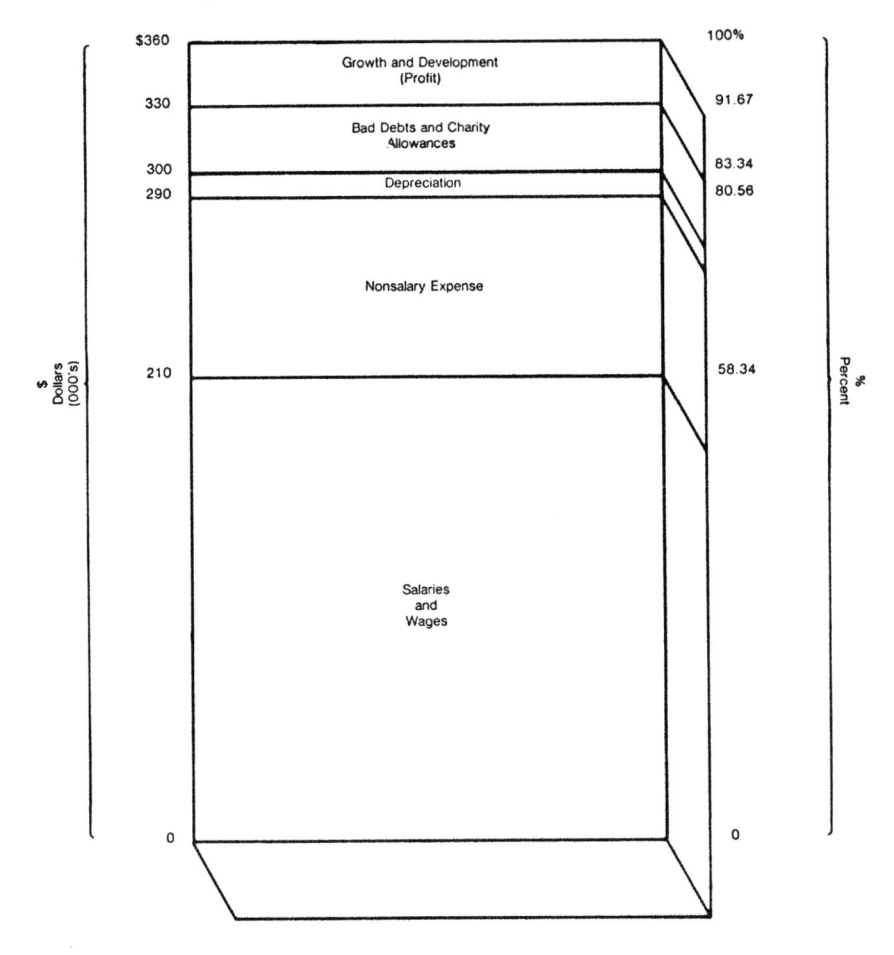

$ Dollars (000's)	Category	% Percent
$360		100%
330	Growth and Development (Profit)	91.67
300	Bad Debts and Charity Allowances	83.34
290	Depreciation	80.56
210	Nonsalary Expense	58.34
0	Salaries and Wages	0

These amounts are illustrated in Figure 9–2. Looking at this illustration, it is easy to see how the burden is shifted from the patient with cost-based coverage who pays $300 per patient day to the full-charge patient who pays $420 per patient day.

As the next step in the case study, assume that the patient mix at Memorial Hospital is as follows:

Patient Description	Number	Percent
Full-Charge	250	25%
Cost-Based	500	50%
80% of Cost	250	25%
Total Patients	1,000	100%

Although the hospital's total financial requirements remain the same, the costs would be distributed as follows:

Description	Full-Charge Patient	Cost-Pay Patient	80% of Cost-Pay Patient	Total
Number of Patients	250	500	250	1,000
Direct Costs				
Salary and Wages	$52,500	$105,000	$52,500	$210,000
Nonsalary Expenses	20,000	40,000	20,000	80,000
Depreciation	2,500	5,000	2,500	10,000
Total Direct Costs	$75,000	$150,000	$75,000	$300,000
Less:				
(a) Provision for Bad Debts and Charity	$30,000	None	None	$30,000
(b) Growth and Development	30,000	None	None	30,000
(c) Loss on 80% Patients	15,000	None	(15,000)	
Total Financial Requirements	$150,000	$150,000	$60,000	$360,000
Average per Patient Day	$600	$300	$240	$360

Figure 9-2 Comparison of Hospital's Average Charge per Patient Day with 50 Percent (500) Cost-Based Patients, Memorial Hospital, Anytown, U.S.A.

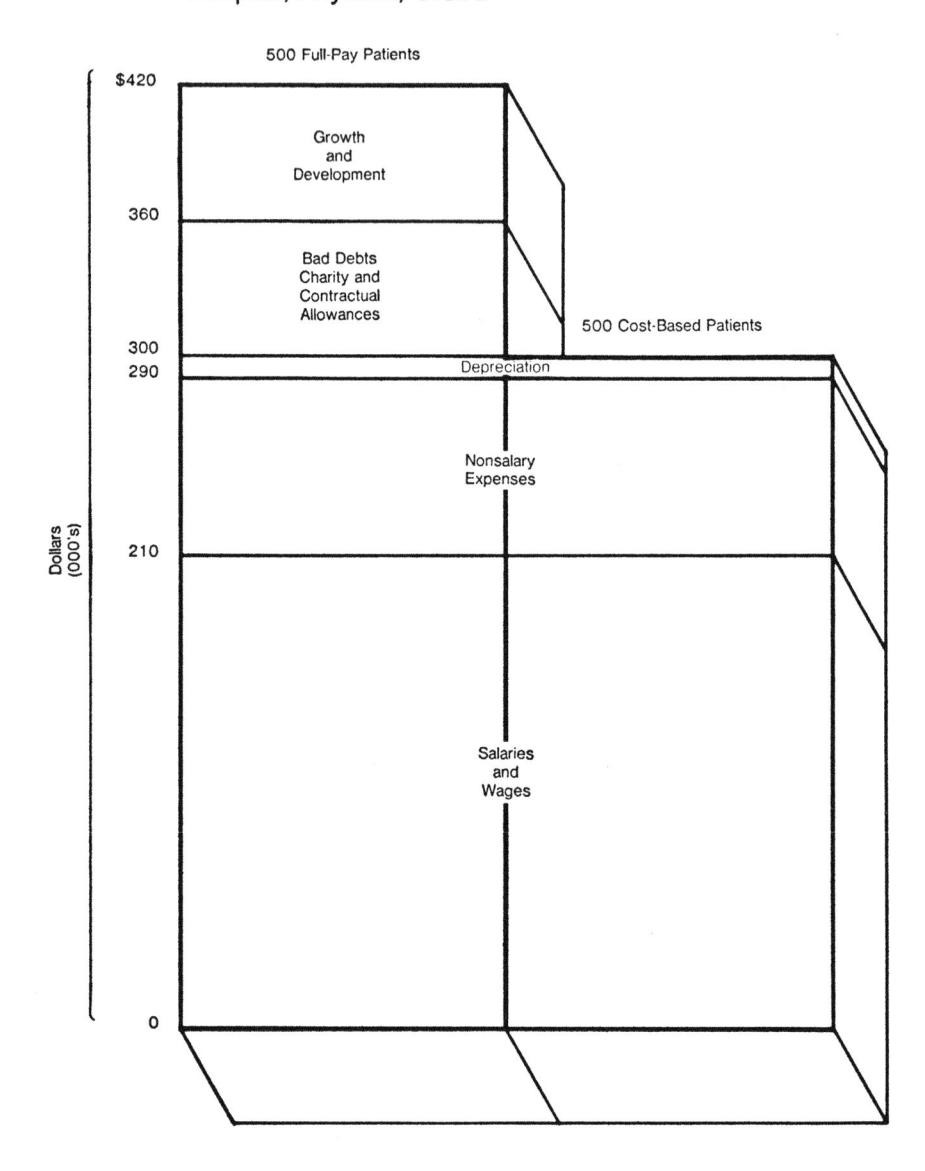

These amounts are illustrated in Figure 9-3. As shown, the burden of meeting the hospital's financial requirements for revenue losses and growth has been shifted more markedly to the full-charge patient. The full-charge patient is charged an average cost of $600 per patient day; the cost-based patient, $300 per day; and the 80 percent of cost-based patient, $240 per day.

Reimbursement under the conditions illustrated in this case study goes far beyond the original congressional intent of the Medicare program. Congress intended that the Medicare program would pay:[10]

- all costs of program beneficiaries and none of nonbeneficiaries
- actual costs, however widely they may vary from one institution to another, unless such costs (in the aggregate) are substantially in excess of those costs incurred by similarly situated institutions in the same area

From these statements, one can infer that Congress did not intend to impose additional "social costs" upon the nonprogram patients.

The Washington State Hospital Commission takes a substantially different position from the third party reimbursement position. The commission states that approved rates should reflect the true financial requirements of each hospital in order to maintain the financial viability of all hospitals. The financial requirements identified by the commission include approved operating expenses, deductions from revenues, that is, bad debts and charity allowances, and an allowance for growth and development. Included in growth and development are elements such as:[11]

- net increases in working capital
- funds for feasibility studies and planning for shared services, mergers, changes in services, expansion, and new equipment

In recognizing the need for growth and development (profit), the state of Washington offers a much more equitable approach to third party reimbursement than either the Medicare or Medicaid programs as they are presently structured.

From 1978 through 1980, the Washington State Hospital Commission, in cooperation with Medicare and Medicaid, conducted a prospective reimbursement demonstration project to test three different payment systems. These systems were:

Type 1: percentage of budget method
Type 2: percentage of charges method
Type 3: traditional retrospective reimbursement through cost finding procedures

188　Patient Account Management

Figure 9–3 Comparison of Hospital's 25% Average Charge per Patient Day with 50 Percent Cost-Based Patients and 25 Percent at 80% of Cost, Memorial Hospital, Anytown, U.S.A.

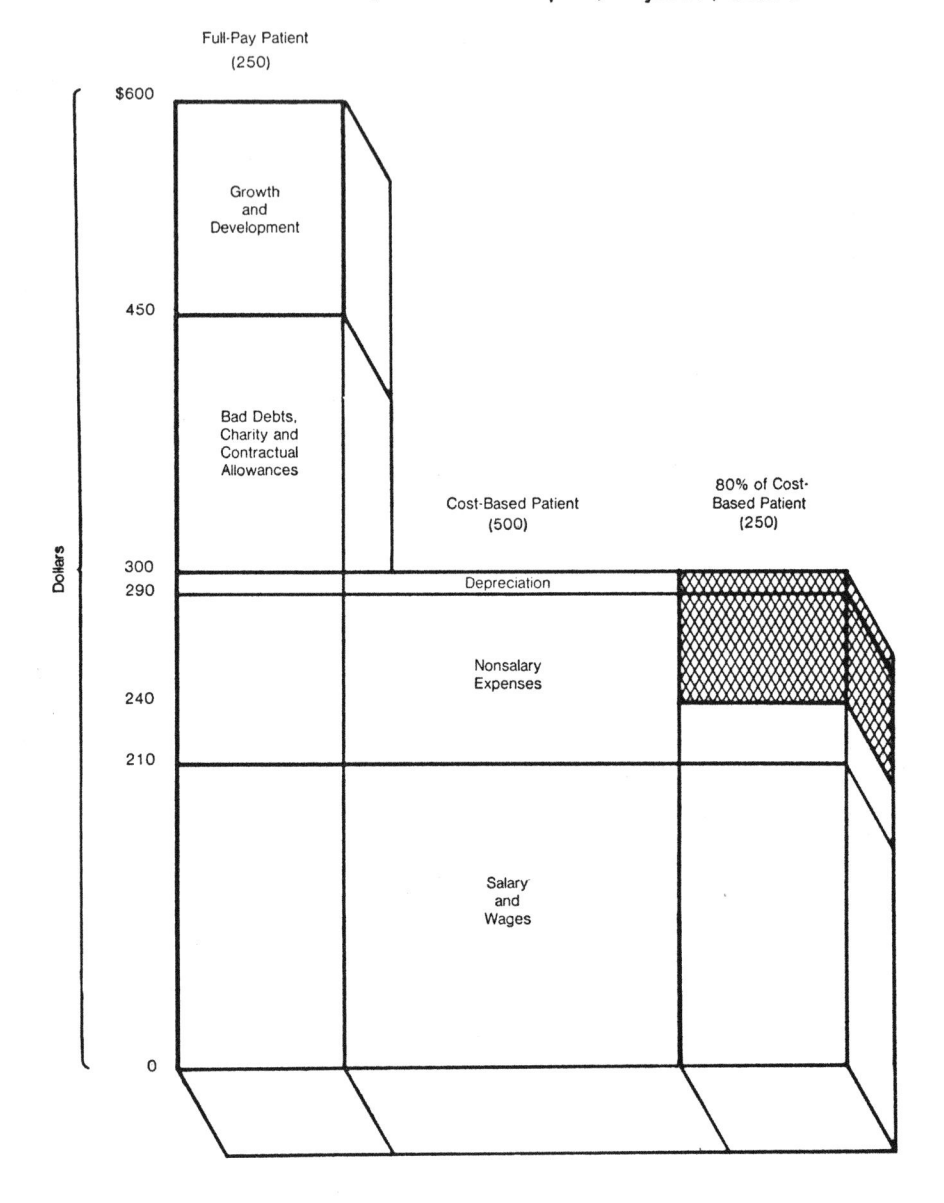

The type 1 payment system was found to be very difficult to administer for both payer and provider. The type 3 payment system, which is not new, of course, proved to be an ineffective system of payment. The type 2 payment system appears to have provided the best results for all concerned. The necessary recordkeeping and accounting for the type 2 payment system proved to be relatively simple for both payer and provider. Furthermore, the results indicated that the cost control incentives inherent in the system were both effective and equitable to all purchasers of services. All payer participants, including Blue Cross, the State Industrial Commission, Medicare, and Medicaid, all paid the same rate. During the first year of the experiment, hospitals reimbursed under the type 1 and type 2 payment systems reduced their rates by five to six percent because the contractual allowances to participating payers were reduced as part of the methodology used. This, of course, meant that charges to all purchasers of service were equitable. As a result, the second year's rates were increased by only three to five percent rather than by the eight to ten percent dictated by general inflation. Unfortunately, even though the Washington research demonstrated that the type 2 payment system would benefit Medicare, Medicaid hospitals and virtually all of the private sector, the experiment was not continued, and the type 2 payment system was never implemented. At the end of the project, inequity in charges and payment continued to exist and seemed likely to even increase.[12]

The Washington experiment has been described here to gain some insight into activities that are being conducted to improve the reimbursement system. The financial officers of the nation's hospitals are the key to the reimbursement dilemma. They must lobby aggressively and protect the financial viability of not only their own hospitals but also the total hospital industry. To do that, hospitals and their financial officers must:

- establish charges based on total financial requirements
- challenge third party interpretation of reimbursement regulations when appropriate
- keep abreast of pending or proposed changes in reimbursement regulations
- become actively involved in trade associations such as the American Hospital Association, the Federation of American Hospitals, and other organizations that are politically active in an effort to keep the institutions that make up the hospital industry viable

In the end, the issue boils down to a simple fact: a hospital is not only a financial business, it is also part of a political process.

RATE SETTING

Rate setting is the process a hospital uses to establish the "price" or "published charge" for the services it provides. Rate setting may be accomplished in two ways:

1. all-inclusive rate: one rate that includes all the services the patient receives during a specific period of time (per patient day), or for a specific condition (per diagnosis)
2. a la carte rate: a rate for every service the patient receives, for example, chest x-ray, blood count, and room and board

The all-inclusive rate is occasionally used in municipal hospitals and long-term health care facilities. As defined above, a single rate per patient day or per diagnosis includes all the services the patient receives as part of that unit. The following example shows how the all-inclusive rate is determined:

Hospital Divisions	Costs
General services	$1,500,000
Financial services	1,000,000
Nursing services	3,000,000
Professional services	2,500,000
Total hospital costs	$8,000,000
Total patient days	20,000
All-inclusive rate per patient day	$ 400
Number of admissions	4,000

If the all-inclusive rate is based upon the number of admissions or diagnoses, the rate would be computed as follows:

$$\frac{\text{Total hospital costs}}{\text{Number of relevant admissions}} = \text{Rate per admission}$$

or

$$\frac{\$8,000,000}{4,000} = \$2,000$$

The all-inclusive rate has these advantages:

- Before admission and/or discharge, the hospital and the patient know how much total patient charges are.

- The charging and accounting systems are relatively simple and easy to understand and compute.
- The charge system facilitates the cash collection process.

Some of the disadvantages of the all-inclusive rate are:

- It does not necessarily represent the amount of financial resources necessary to produce the service.
- It does not produce a system conducive to the price sensitivity testing necessary to ensure profitability.

In most instances, the disadvantages of the all-inclusive rate far outweigh the advantages.

The a la carte system of rate setting is the most common method used in the hospital industry. The key to a la carte rate setting is the selection of the unit of service to be priced. Units of service may be either macro or micro. The macro unit of service is one that grossly represents the service a patient receives, for example, x-ray examination, laboratory test, and operating room care. Even though this statistic has considerable value, it does not adequately represent the amount of resources the hospital used to furnish the service.

The micro unit of service endeavors to establish a series of relative value units (RVUs) for each service. The value assigned to each RVU is directly proportional to the amount of resources, that is, labor, supplies, and equipment, required to provide the service. The most commonly used relative value unit system is the workload measurement for laboratory services developed by the College of American Pathologists (CAP). Under this system, the hospital can determine a price per RVU and simply multiply this price (charge) by the number of RVUs assigned to each laboratory test. The RVU cost is computed as follows:

Laboratory

Description	Total Cost	Unit Cost
Direct Expenses		
Salaries and Wages	$ 800,000	$ .40
Nonsalary Expense	600,000	.30
Depreciation	200,000	.10
Total Direct Expense	$1,600,000	$ .80
Plus: Allocated Costs	800,000	.40
Total Accounting Costs	$2,400,000	$1.20

Laboratory

Description	Total Cost	Unit Cost
Plus: Provision for		
(a) Deduction	$ 240,000	$ .12
(b) Profit	240,000	.12
Total Economic Costs	$2,880,000	$1.44
Total Relative Value Units	2,000,000	1

Whichever rate setting methodology the hospital adopts, it is important to test its price sensitivity to the third party reimbursement system. Usually, it is not in the hospital's best interest to use a common profit margin for all departments. Each revenue-producing department should be analyzed in order to determine the percent of charges generated by the third party cost-based payer. As a general rule, departments that provide the largest portion of services to a cost-based payer should have a narrow profit margin. That reduces the amount to be written off as a contractual allowance. Conversely, revenue-generating departments with lower utilization by cost-based programs should have a broader profit margin to maximize the cash flow from charge-based patients. The following example illustrates this rate setting policy.

Assume that Memorial Hospital's laboratory and radiology departments have identified these operating expenses:

	Laboratory	*Radiology*
Direct Expenses	$1,600,000	$1,600,000
Allocated Expenses	800,000	800,000
Total Expense	$2,400,000	$2,400,000

If a uniform profit margin of 25 percent is applied to the total expenses, the planned profit would be $600,000.

Assume that 60 percent of laboratory services and 30 percent of radiology services were purchased by cost-based programs. The comparative operating statement would be:

	Laboratory	*Radiology*
Cost-based Reimbursement	60%	30%
Revenue:	$3,000,000	$3,000,000
(@ 25% Total Expense)		
Less: Contractual Allowances	360,000	180,000
Net Revenue	$2,640,000	$2,820,000
Total Expense	$2,400,000	$2,400,000
Net Profit	$240,000	$420,000

Instead of using the common 25 percent profit margin on total expenses, the laboratory margin can be reduced to 15 percent and the radiology margin can be increased to 30 percent, with these results:

	Laboratory	Radiology
Cost-based Reimbursement	60%	30%
Revenue:		
(a) 15% on Expenses	$2,760,000	
(b) 30% on Expenses		$3,168,000
Less: Contractual Allowances	$216,000	230,400
Net Revenue	$2,544,000	$2,937,600
Total Expense	$2,400,000	$2,400,000
Net Profit	$144,000	$537,600

The uniform and nonuniform markup systems can be compared as follows:

	Uniform	Nonuniform	Variance
Contractual Allowances:			
Laboratory	$360,000	$216,000	$(144,000)
Radiology	180,000	230,400	50,400
Total	$540,000	$446,400	$ (93,600)
Net Profits:			
Laboratory	$240,000	$144,000	$ (96,000)
Radiology	420,000	$537,600	117,600
Total	$660,000	$681,600	$ 21,600

By decreasing the uniform markup percentage from 25 percent to 15 percent for the laboratory and increasing it to 30 percent for the radiology department, the hospital can:

- reduce total contractual allowances by $93,600—from $540,000 to $464,400
- increase total net profits (potential cash flow) by $21,600—from $660,000 to $681,600

This illustration underscores the importance of establishing a rate setting policy that is sensitive to the methods third party payers use to reimburse hospitals.

In summary, it is absolutely necessary to use price sensitivity testing on a departmental basis. The ideal hospital rate setting policy should emphasize:

- reducing the amount of contractual allowances
- maximizing cash inflows
- obtaining a reasonable profit

The patient account manager should be acutely aware of the pricing techniques and objectives such as those described and should be prepared to assist management in attaining these objectives. The patient account manager must know the hospital's method of determining prices for services to be able to explain clearly to the troubled or puzzled patient how and why these charges are established.

By being keenly aware of rate setting techniques, the patient account manager can better serve the patient as well as the hospital. The patient account manager can no longer afford to sit on the sidelines when rates and reimbursement are determined; he/she must be involved.

NOTES

1. *Factors to Evaluate in the Establishment of Hospital Charges* (Chicago: American Hospital Association), p. 10.
2. Howard J. Berman and Lewis E. Weeks, *The Financial Management of Hospitals* (Ann Arbor, Mich.: Health Administration Press, 1976), p. 206.
3. Ibid. p. 178.
4. L. Vann Seawell, *Hospital Financial Accounting Theory and Practice* (Chicago: Hospital Financial Management Association, 1975), p. 198.
5. Peter F. Drucker, *Management: Tasks, Responsibilities, and Practices* (New York: Harper & Row, 1974), pp. 98–99.
6. Peter F. Drucker, *Managing in Turbulent Times* (New York: Harper & Row, 1980), p. 31.
7. Ibid., pp. 33–34.
8. Ibid., p. 34.
9. Ibid., pp. 34–35.
10. "Medicare Reimbursement," Jack C. Wood, ed., *Topics in Health Care Financing* 1, no. 3 (Spring 1975): 8.
11. Frank D. Baker, "Prospective Rate Setting," William L. Dowling, ed., *Topics in Health Care Financing* 3, no. 2 (Winter 1976): 59–60.
12. Clarence F. Legel, *The Washington State Hospital Commission Prospective Reimbursement Demonstration Project* (Spokane, Wash.: Unpublished report, 1981).

Chapter 10

Cash Forecasting and Management

Cash forecasting and management is an integral part of the hospital's budgetary control system. The budgetary control system begins with the preparation of the operating budget and capital expenditure plans. Once they have been completed, cash forecasting and management can begin.

The first step in cash forecasting is to analyze the monthly income and expense statements to determine cash inflows and outflows. The time lag factors explained below are used in this analysis. In reality, cash forecasting turns the hospital's accrual system into a cash accounting statement.

Basically, two time lag factors must be computed and monitored:

1. cash inflow time lag factor: the amount of time between billing of the patient for services and receipt of payment by the hospital
2. cash outflow time lag factor: the amount of time between the incurring of an expense by the hospital and actual disbursement of cash to pay it

Management can control each time lag factor with any one of several methods, each of which features varying degrees of efficiency. Techniques for matching cash inflows and outflows for the most appropriate and profitable use of the hospital's resources will be discussed later in this chapter.

PURPOSE

The primary purpose of cash forecasting and management is to assist management in determining whether there will be enough cash coming in to cover projected expenditures. The forecasting helps prepare management for the fact that additional funds may be needed to carry out the operating budget and the capital expenditure plan. The process also alerts management to the existence of surplus operating funds that can be invested, thus allowing the hospital to maximize its cash resources.

A secondary purpose of cash forecasting and management is to help the hospital satisfy the requirement of the Joint Commission on Accreditation of Hospitals (JCAH) that the hospital chief executive officer (CEO), consistent with governing board policy, maintain and safeguard appropriate physical resources and use them judiciously to implement hospital programs and meet patient needs. JCAH also prescribes that the CEO be responsible for implementing governing board policy covering the financial management of the hospital. This includes the development of cash inflow budgets.[1]

Effective cash forecasting and management will help ensure that the hospital has enough cash to:

- meet operating needs
- finance capital expenditures
- receive maximum earnings from investments

Basically, there are five ways to increase cash resources:

1. reduce the amount of current assets, for example, accounts receivable, inventories, and prepaid expenses
2. increase the amount of current liabilities, for example, accounts payable
3. increase operating revenues, that is, charges to patients, and reduce operating expenses
4. restrict capital expenditures
5. use bank float

These techniques can be used independently or combined. The first four are self-explanatory; use of bank float will be discussed later in this chapter.

If the hospital has a reasonably steady or even inflow of cash, its ideal operating cash balance is zero. A zero balance means that management is indeed using the hospital's resources judiciously.

MAJOR COMPONENTS

The cash forecasting and management process involves the control of four major components:

- cash inflows
- cash outflows

- borrowings and investments
- bank float

Cash inflows, cash outflows, and borrowings and investments are all shown in the cash forecast statement. Bank float, on the other hand, is not shown on the statement because it represents cash available only for a very limited time.

Cash Inflows

Patient accounts receivable usually represent a hospital's largest asset and its greatest source of cash inflows. There are two bases for forecasting cash from patient revenue:

1. gross charges to patients
2. net charges to patients

The basic distinction between the two is that the gross amount is determined before adjustments for deductions, for example, bad debts, contractual allowances, and courtesy discounts, have been applied. Net charges are determined after these deductions have been made. There are conflicting opinions about which method is better. In this book, the net charges method is preferred, and it will be the approach described in this chapter.

Borrowings, or outside financing, for example, loans, mortgages, bonds, and stock issues, constitute the hospital's second largest source of cash inflows. Short-term loan and investment accounts are frequently used in the cash inflow statement as balancing accounts to show additional funds generated from short-term loans or the investment of surplus cash. The cash inflows from borrowings and investments are entered in the master cash forecast statement as shown in Table 10–1, line 2c.

The remaining cash inflows to the hospital usually come from a variety of sources including:

- cafeteria sales
- medical record transcription
- investment income
- transfer from other hospital funds
- rentals
- vendors
- concessions
- gifts and donations
- other nonpatient revenue

198 PATIENT ACCOUNT MANAGEMENT

Table 10–1 Master Cash Forecast Statement

Memorial Hospital, Anytown, U.S.A.
Master Cash Forecast Statement
For the Budget Year Ending December 31, 19x1
(in thousands of dollars)

	1	2	3	4	5	6	7	8	9	10	11	12	Total
1. Beginning cash balance	$ 50	$ 0	$ 0	$ 0	$ 0	$ 0	$ 0	$ 0	$ 0	$ 0	$ 0	$ 0	$ 50
2. Cash Inflows:													
a. Net patient receivables	$227	$277	$287	$308	$316	$327	$326	$323	$316	$302	$313	$320	$3,642
b. Other operating sources	20	13	16	21	16	14	15	15	14	20	16	26	206
c. Borrowings (investments)	(28)	(39)	(26)	(51)	(50)	32	39	(9)	52	(33)	(38)	51	(100)
d. Total cash inflows	$219	$251	$277	$278	$282	$373	$380	$329	$382	$289	$291	$397	$3,748
3. Total cash-on-hand (line 1 + line 2 = line 3)	$269	$251	$277	$278	$282	$373	$380	$329	$382	$289	$291	$397	$3,798
4. Cash Outflows:													
a. Salary, wages, and related expenses	$190	$184	$196	$193	$198	$197	$201	$199	$203	$198	$204	$205	$2,368
b. Capital expenditures	5	0	10	0	5	100	100	50	100	10	5	110	495
c. Noncapital, nonsalary expenses	74	67	71	85	79	76	79	80	79	81	82	82	935
d. Total cash outflows	$269	$251	$277	$278	$282	$373	$380	$329	$382	$289	$291	$397	$3,798
5. Ending cash balance (line 3 − line 4 = line 5)	$-0-	$-0-	$-0-	$-0-	$-0-	$-0-	$-0-	$-0-	$-0-	$-0-	$-0-	$-0-	$-0-

It may be noted here that some hospitals have found fund-raising drives to be an excellent source of cash, while others have not. To gauge whether the hospital should undertake a fund-raising drive, hospital management must consider the community and its likely response to a campaign for gifts.

Cash Outflows

Basically, cash outflows can be divided into three major classifications:

1. salary, wages, and other related expenses
2. programmed nonsalary expenses
3. variable nonsalary expenses

A hospital's largest cash outflow is for salary, wages, and related expenses, for example, social security taxes, retirement benefits, and group insurance premiums. Although these expenses are usually budgeted on a monthly basis, for cash management purposes, they must be planned according to the frequency of actual cash disbursement to the employee, whether it be weekly, biweekly, or monthly.

Programmed nonsalary expenses are those for which payment is scheduled or programmed for specific times throughout the year. Such expenses include:

- insurance premiums
- capital expenditures
- mortgage payments
- short-term loans
- rentals and leases
- utilities

Except for utilities, programmed expenses represent a fixed amount of money that does not vary regardless of volume of activity. Capital expenditures are handled as a separate line item direct from the capital budget.

Variable nonsalary expenses are operating expenses, for example, medical and surgical supplies and office supplies, that vary in direct proportion to the volume of work.

In one way or another, all the expenses or purchases in the hospital's revenue and expense statement and capital expenditure plan are recorded in its cash forecast, except the provision for depreciation. Depreciation is a noncash item that must be included in computing the hospital's total operating expenses. Since depreciation is really an accounting device to indicate the amortization of a capital purchase, it is not included in the cash forecast. A capital expenditure is recorded in the cash forecast only when cash is actually paid out, or when the payment of that cash is planned.

Borrowings and Investments

Borrowings and/or investments are usually shown as a balancing account in a cash forecast. For example, after all cash inflows and outflows have been computed for the month, the cash forecaster may find that cash inflows are not sufficient to cover cash outflows. In this case, the required cash must be borrowed to maintain the necessary bank balance. On the other hand, if the cash forecaster finds that cash available to the hospital after cash outflows have been taken into account is too great to remain in a noninterest-bearing checking account, the surplus will be invested.

There are two commonly used methods for recording these activities. In the first method, each activity is considered a separate function or account. Therefore, borrowings would be considered cash inflows and investments would be treated as cash outflows.

The second method considers these two activities as a single line item under cash inflows. If cash is borrowed, the amount would be recorded in the same manner as any other cash inflow. If cash is invested, the amount would be bracketed as illustrated below:

	January	February	March	Total
Borrowings (investments)	$10,000	$20,000	($15,000)	$15,000

An advantage of using one line item is that the balancing account can be identified quickly because it is netted out in the total column. Moreover, using two line items requires an additional computation.

Bank Float

Bank float represents an intangible and relatively uncontrollable amount of cash that the hospital can use by taking advantage of cash in transit. Bank float represents the portion of the bank balance created by the time interval between the drawing of checks on the hospital's account and the actual debiting of the account for those checks. Positive float allows the hospital to operate with a book balance that is actually less than the compensating balance the bank requires the hospital to maintain.[2] For example, if a hospital generally has $100,000 in outstanding checks at the time the bank account balance is reconciled to the hospital bank balance, this amount could be used for short-term investments or for payment of additional expenses. One word of caution about the use of bank float is absolutely necessary: it requires relatively constant and consistent cash flow.

CASH FORECASTING METHODOLOGY

As stated earlier, the hospital's operating budget and capital expenditure plan must be completed before cash forecasting, that is, the analysis of time-lag factors and amounts of cash inflows and outflows can begin. The two major analyses involved in cash forecasting are:

1. cash receipts analysis
2. cash disbursement analysis

Cash Receipts Analysis

The first step in cash forecasting is to analyze cash inflows from patient accounts receivable. This analysis involves determining:

- the type of paying agent
- the length of time before payment

Assume that the analysis of gross charges to patients indicates that the mix of paying agents corresponds to the one shown in Table 10–2.

Historical cash receipts are then analyzed and time lag factors are established for each paying agent based on the amount of time it takes to collect cash from that agent for services rendered. Generally, the accounts

Table 10–2 Percent Analysis of Gross Charges to Patients by Paying Agent, Memorial Hospital, Anytown, U.S.A.

Paying Agent	% of Gross Charges
Blue Cross	30%
Medicare	40
Medicaid	10
Commercial Insurance	15
Self-Pay and Others	5
Total	100%

of most patients are not paid in full with a single payment; rather the payment period may extend over time. For example, assume that a patient with commercial insurance has a $5,000 account. The payoff schedule might look like this:

Time of Payment	Source of Payment	Amount of Payment (Dollars)	(Percents)
Admissions day	Patient deposit	$ 500	10%
30 days after billing	Insurance	$3,600	72%
60 days after billing	Patient	$ 450	9%
90 days after billing	Patient	$ 450	9%
Total		$5,000	100%

The process of analyzing each paying agent's payment schedule is extremely time consuming. In addition, these schedules can vary according to outside economic factors such as inflation and high interest rates. For this reason, the patient account manager should conduct only a statistical sampling of the process instead of using a large amount of hours and resources to do a comprehensive study. The best approach is to do a periodic statistical sampling of payment schedules and time lag factors purely for verification and control.

The second step in cash forecasting is analysis of cash inflows from gross charges to patients according to the time cash is received. Table 10–3 shows a typical mix of payment schedules and time lag factors by paying agent. It should be noted that paying agents are classified into major groups in the table. However, some patient account managers might find it beneficial

Table 10–3 Percent Analysis of Cash Payment Schedules and Time Lag Factors of Gross Charges to Patients by Paying Agent, Memorial Hospital, Anytown, U.S.A.

Paying Agent	1	2	3	4	5	6	7	Total %
Blue Cross	50	30	15	5	—	—	—	100%
Medicare	60	25	10	5	—	—	—	100
Medicaid	10	20	30	20	10	5	5	100
Commercial Insurance	30	40	15	10	5	—	—	100
Self-Pay and Others	15	25	25	15	10	5	5	100

% of Payments Schedule Month After Charges Are Generated

to expand these classifications, especially if some categories include agents with widely different reimbursement systems or payment schedules. For example, a hospital may be a member of two Blue Cross plans, one of which pays the hospital prospectively based on patient gross charges, while the other pays the hospital based on costs with a retroactive adjustment based at the end of the fiscal period. Another good reason for a more detailed breakdown of paying agents would be the need for closer surveillance of cash inflows in situations in which one commercial insurance company or health maintenance organization (HMO) dominates its segment of the market.

After payment schedules and time lag factors have been analyzed by paying agent, the next step is to determine the net charges to patients by making provisions for contractual allowances and bad debts for each paying agent as illustrated in Table 10–4.

Basically, there are two different methods used to forecast cash inflows from paying agents. One is the weighted average monthly cash inflow percentage method, which relies on a weighted average such as the one illustrated in Table 10–5.[3]

The following formula is used in the weighted average computation:

Let:

MC = Monthly collection percentage
R = Revenue percentage
$(R \times MC^1)$ = Weighted percentage (first month)
$\Sigma(R \times MC^1)$ = Sum total of weighted percentage (first month)

In this illustration, the sum of the weighted averages $\Sigma(R \times MC^1)$ for the first month is computed as follows:

Table 10–4 Percent Analysis of Net Patient Charges by Paying Agents, Memorial Hospital, Anytown, U.S.A.

Paying Agent	Gross Charges	Less: Provision for Deductibles	Net Charges
Blue Cross	100%	10%	90%
Medicare	100	20	80
Medicaid	100	40	60
Commercial Insurance	100	5	95
Self-Pay and Others	100	15	85

Table 10-5 Analysis and Computation of Weighted Collection Percentage of Patient Charges Collected, Memorial Hospital, Anytown, U.S.A.

Paying Agent	R % of Total Revenue	First MC¹	R×MC¹	Second MC²	R×MC²	Third MC³	R×MC³	Fourth MC⁴	R×MC⁴	Fifth MC⁵	R×MC⁵	Sixth MC⁶	R×MC⁶	Seventh MC⁷	R×MC⁷
Blue Cross	30%	50	15.0	30	9.0	15	4.5	5	1.5	—	—	—	—	—	—
Medicare	40	60	24.0	25	10.0	10	4.0	5	2.0	—	—	—	—	—	—
Medicaid	10	10	1.0	20	2.0	30	3.0	20	2.0	10	1.0	5	.5	5	.5
Commercial Insurance	15	30	4.5	40	6.0	15	2.3	10	1.5	5	.8	—	—	—	—
Self-Pay and Others	5	15	.8	25	1.2	25	1.2	15	.8	10	.5	5	.2	5	.2
Total Σ(R × MC)	100%		45.3		28.2		15.0		7.8		2.3		.7		.7

Paying Agent	$(R \times MC^1)$
Blue Cross	15.0%
Medicare	24.0
Medicaid	1.0
Commercial Insurance	4.5
Self-Pay and Others	0.8
Total	45.3%

This means that 45.3 percent of total patient charges should be collected in cash during the first month after these charges are generated. A complete cash collection schedule of patient charges is shown in Table 10–6.

The second method used to forecast cash inflows from patient charges is to analyze the cash inflows by paying agent. If a computer is available, this method is recommended because of its greater accuracy. However, if the cash forecast is to be done manually, the weighted average method is preferable. Table 10–7 is an example of an application of the weighted average percentage developed in Table 10–6.

Table 10–7 starts with the beginning patient accounts receivable balance of $500,000, which is distributed by the weighted average collection method. Net charges to patients are distributed on a monthly basis and totaled for each month as the cash inflows from net patient charges for that month. Any uncollected net charges are accumulated in the far right-hand column to determine the ending patient accounts receivable balance for the period.

The cash inflows from other operating sources, such as cafeteria sales and medical records transcriptions, are then analyzed as illustrated in Table 10–8, and the total is spread on the master cash flow statement (see Table 10–1, line 2b, page 198). The next step is to enter the cash inflows from

Table 10–6 Weighted Average Cash Collection Schedule of Patient Charges, Memorial Hospital, Anytown, U.S.A.

Month After Charges Are Generated	Weighted Average Collected
1	45.3%
2	28.2%
3	15.0%
4	7.8%
5	2.3%
6	.7%
7	.7%
Total	100.0%

206   PATIENT ACCOUNT MANAGEMENT

Table 10-7 Cash Inflow Analysis of Net Patient Charges

Memorial Hospital, Anytown, U.S.A.
Cash Inflow Analysis of Net Patient Charges
For the Budget Year Ending December 31, 19x1
(in thousands of dollars)

Month	Beginning Patient Accounts Receivable Balance	1	2	3	4	5	6	7	8	9	10	11	12	Ending Patient Accounts Receivable Balance
1	$500	(45.3) $227	(28.2) $141	(15.0) $75	(7.8) $39	(2.3) $12	(.7) $3	(.7) $3						
2	300		136	85	45	23	7	2	$2					
3	280			127	79	42	22	6	2	$2				
4	320				145	90	48	25	8	2	$2			
5	330					149	93	49	27	8	2	$2		
6	340						154	96	51	27	8	2	$2	
7	320							145	90	48	25	8	2	$2
8	315								143	89	47	25	7	4
9	310									140	87	47	24	12
10	290										131	82	44	33
11	325											147	92	86
12	330												149	181
														310
Total net charges to patients	$3,770													
Cash inflow from net charges	$3,642	$227	$277	$287	$308	$316	$327	$326	$323	$316	$302	$313	$320	
Ending patient accounts receivable balance														$628

Note: Net charges were distributed using the weighted average collection in Table 10–6.

Table 10–8 Analysis of Monthly Cash Inflows from Other Operating Sources

Memorial Hospital, Anytown, U.S.A.
Analysis of Monthly Cash Inflows from Other Operating Sources
For the Budget Year Ending December 31, 19x1
(in thousands of dollars)

Month	Cafeteria	Medical Records	Other	Total
1	$ 10	$ 2	$ 8	$ 20
2	8	1	4	13
3	9	1	6	16
4	11	2	8	21
5	10	1	5	16
6	9	1	4	14
7	8	1	6	15
8	9	2	4	15
9	10	1	3	14
10	9	2	9	20
11	10	2	4	16
12	10	1	15	26
Total	$113	$17	$76	$206

net patient receivables in the master cash flow statement (see Table 10–1, line 2a, page 198). Once these inflows have been recorded, the analysis of cash outflows can begin.

Cash Disbursement Analysis

As stated earlier, cash outflows must be handled on a cash basis, even though the hospital uses the accrual accounting method. Generally, hospitals have a separate imprest fund for processing payroll checks. In that case, the hospital may transfer an amount equal to the net amount of the payroll from the general operating fund to the imprest payroll account. Separate checks to cover payroll taxes and related expenses are also drawn on the operating fund for deposit in the imprest payroll account.

Another way of handling an imprest payroll account is to deposit an amount equal to the total payroll, including the amount withheld from employees for taxes and other withholding requirements, in the imprest payroll account. There are many ways a hospital can use imprest payroll accounts. However, some hospitals do not use imprest payroll accounts at all, simply disbursing payroll from the general operating fund. Nevertheless, salary, wages, and related expenses must be shown on the cash forecast statement at the time payroll checks are disbursed.

Most hospitals disburse payroll and related expenses in the month in which they are budgeted. Within that month, however, there is a time lag between disbursement of the check to the employee and the cashing of that check. A typical time lag factor is shown in Table 10–9. Note that 30 percent of the hospital's employees cash their payroll checks on payday, while 5 percent of the employees cash their checks as long as 23 to 30 days after they are issued. The hospital can use the kind of information shown in Table 10–9 to make short-term investments by staggering payments from the general operating fund to the imprest payroll account to cover payroll checks as they are cashed.

For illustration, assume that Memorial Hospital of Anytown, U.S.A. pays its employees on the first and fifteenth of each month. Assume further that the cash outflows for salary, wages, and related expenses for Memorial Hospital's budget year ending December 31, 19x1 are as shown in Table 10–10. (These cash outflows are shown on the master cash flow statement in Table 10–1, line 4a, page 198).

Nonsalary cash outflows can be divided into two major categories of expenditure:

1. capital
2. noncapital

Table 10–9 Analysis of Employee Payroll Cashing Process, Memorial Hospital, Anytown, U.S.A.

Number of Days After Issuance	Amount Dollar	%	Employees Number	%
1	$21,375	25%	195	30%
2	12,825	15	130	20
3	8,550	10	98	15
4	8,550	10	65	10
5	6,840	8	52	8
6	1,710	2	13	2
7	8,550	10	39	6
8–14	4,275	5	13	2
15–22	4,275	5	13	2
23–30	8,550	10	32	5
Total	$85,500	100%	650	100%

Table 10-10 Analysis of Cash Outflow for Salary, Wages, and Related Expenses

Memorial Hospital, Anytown, U.S.A.
Analysis of Cash Outflow for Salary, Wages, and Related Expenses
For the Budget Year Ending December 31, 19x1
(in thousands of dollars)

Month	Payroll Date	Monthly Payroll	Payroll Related Expense	Total Salary, Wages, and Related Expenses
1	1/1– 1/15	$ 165	$ 25	$ 190
2	2/1– 2/15	160	24	184
3	3/1– 3/15	170	26	196
4	4/1– 4/15	118	25	193
5	5/1– 5/15	172	26	198
6	6/1– 6/15	170	27	197
7	7/1– 7/15	175	26	201
8	8/1– 8/15	173	26	199
9	9/1– 9/15	176	27	203
10	10/1–10/15	172	26	198
11	11/1–11/15	177	27	204
12	12/1–12/15	178	27	205
Total		$2,056	$312	$2,368

Cash outflows for capital expenditures come directly from the hospital's capital expenditure plan or capital budget. For illustration, Memorial Hospital's capital expenditure plan for the budget year ending December 31, 19x1 is shown in Table 10–11. (These totals are recorded on the master cash flow statement in Table 10–1, line 4b, page 198).

Noncapital cash outflows can be classified by several methods. For purposes of this discussion, these expenditures are classified as either:

- programmed
- variable

Programmed expenditures are those noncapital, nonsalary cash flow requirements such as:

- utilities
- rent and/or leases
- insurance
- mortgage payments

210 PATIENT ACCOUNT MANAGEMENT

Table 10–11 Summary Analysis of Capital Expenditure Cash Flow Requirements

Memorial Hospital, Anytown, U.S.A.
Summary Analysis of Capital Expenditure Cash Flow Requirements
For the Budget Year Ending December 31, 19x1
(in thousands of dollars)

Month	Amount Needed
1	$ 5
2	-0-
3	10
4	-0-
5	5
6	100
7	100
8	50
9	100
10	10
11	5
12	110
Total	$495

In short, these expenses are fixed payments that are essential in order to provide the facilities and equipment necessary to perform services to patients.

Variable noncapital, nonsalary expenses are those cash outflow requirements that usually vary in direct proportion to the volume of work, that is, patient days and outpatient visits.

Setting priorities for payment of individual expenses is a method used by some hospitals to schedule cash outflows. Table 10–12 shows the payment priority classification system Memorial Hospital uses for all cash outflows. Memorial Hospital has analyzed its noncapital, nonsalary cash outflows as shown in Table 10–13. The accumulated percentages in the right-hand column of Table 10–14 are then applied to the hospital's budgeted noncapital, nonsalary expenses shown in Table 10–15. The monthly cash outflows for these expenses are then recorded in the master cash flow statement (see Table 10–1, line 4c, page 198).

At the beginning of the cash forecasting process, the cash balance was $50,000 (see Table 10–1, line 1, page 198). During the first month, the total cash inflows shown in Table 10–1 were:

Table 10–12 Payment Priority Classification for Cash Outflows, Memorial Hospital, Anytown, U.S.A.

Payment Priority	Description of Payment	Payment Schedules from Date of Receipt
A	Payroll, Commission, etc.	Current month
B	Mortgage, Rent, Leases, Utilities, Service Contracts	Current month
C	Foods, Medical and Surgical Supplies, Drugs	30 days (following month)
D	Discount Vendors	30 days (following month)
E	Funded Depreciation, Investments	30 days (following month)
F	Special Vendors	30–59 days (second month)
G	Other Vendors	60–90 days (third month)

Table 10–13 Schedule of Noncapital, Nonsalary Cash Outflow Requirements

Memorial Hospital, Anytown, U.S.A.
Schedule of Noncapital, Nonsalary Cash Outflow Requirements
(in thousands of dollars)

Month	Cash Requirement	1–15 Days A, B = 55%	15–30 Days C = 10%	30 Days D, E = 10%	30–45 Days F = 10%	45–90 Days G = 15%
1	$ 70	$39	$7	$7	$7	$10
2	73	40	7	7	7	12
3	78	43	8	8	8	11
4	77	42	8	8	8	11
5	79	43	8	8	8	12
6	75	41	8	8	8	10
7	80	44	8	8	8	12
8	80	44	8	8	8	12
9	82	45	8	8	8	13
10	81	45	8	8	8	12
11	83	46	8	8	8	13
12	82	45	8	8	8	13
Total	$940					

Table 10-14 Analysis of Noncapital, Nonsalary Cash Outflows by Priority Classification, Memorial Hospital, Anytown, U.S.A.

Priority Classification	Payment Schedule from Date of Receipt	Percent of Cash Outflows	Monthly Accumulated Percentage
A	Current month	40	—
B	Current month	15	55
C	30 days	10	—
D	30 days	5	—
E	30 days	5	75
F	30–59 days	10	85
G	60–90 days	15	100%
Total		100%	

Line

2a	Net patient receivables	$227,000
2b	Other operating revenue	20,000
	Total cash inflows	$247,000

Thus, total cash on hand is $297,000.
Total cash outflows were:

Line

4a	Salary, wages, and related expenses	$190,000
4b	Capital expenditures	5,000
4c	Noncapital, nonsalary expenses	74,000
4d	Total cash outflows	$269,000

Hence, there is a cash net difference or balance of $28,000. Since the hospital had adopted a "zero" cash balance policy, the $28,000 is invested in short-term instruments, leaving a net cash inflow of $219,000 (see Table 10–1, line 2d, page 198) and a total of $269,000 cash on hand for the month. Checking the borrowings/investment account (see Table 10–1, line 2c, page 198), the cash forecaster can project the need to either borrow or invest.

During the second month, $39,000 was deposited in the investment account, representing excess cash inflows. During the following three months,

Table 10-15 Schedule of Noncapital, Nonsalary Cash Outflow Requirements

Memorial Hospital, Anytown, U.S.A.
Schedule of Noncapital, Nonsalary Cash Outflow Requirements
For the Budget Year Ending December 31, 19x1
(in thousands of dollars)

Month	Beginning Accounts Payable Balance	1 (.55)	2 (.75)	3 (.85)	4 (1.00)	5	6	7	8	9	10	11	12	Ending Accounts Payable Balance
1	$65	$35	$13	$7	$10									
2	70	39	14	7	10									
3	73		40	14	7	$12								
4	78			43	16	8	$11							
5	77				42	16	8	$11						
6	79					43	16	8	$12					
7	75						41	16	8	$10				
8	80							44	16	8	$12			
9	80								44	16	8	$12		
10	82									45	16	8	$13	
11	81										46	16	8	$12
12	83											—	16	21
	82												45	37
Total cash requirements	$1,005													
Cash outflow for expenses	$935	$74	$67	$71	$85	$79	$76	$79	$80	$79	$81	$82	$82	
Ending accounts payable balance														$70

the following additions were added to the investment account, making a total of $194,000 in investments:

Month	Amount Deposited
3	$26,000
4	51,000
5	50,000
	$127,000

During the sixth month, the shortfall of cash inflows to cash outflows was $32,000; this amount was withdrawn from the investment account. During the seventh month, there was a $39,000 shortfall. The following is a recalculation of the borrowings/investment account at the end of the seventh month:

Month	Deposits	Withdrawals	Balance
1	$28,000		$ 28,000
2	39,000		67,000
3	26,000		93,000
4	51,000		144,000
5	50,000		194,000
6		$32,000	162,000
7		39,000	123,000

The subsequent months' cash flow forecasts were projected in the same manner, that is, using the borrowings/investment account as the "equalizer." The annual result was a total net cash investment of $100,000 (see Table 10–1, line 2c, page 198). A summary of the budgeted cash inflows and outflows is:

Beginning Cash Balance	$ 50,000
Plus:	
Cash Inflows:	
Net Patient Accounts Receivable	$3,642,000
Other Operating Services	206,000
Total Cash Inflows	$3,848,000
Cash on Hand	$3,898,000

Less:
　Cash Outflows:
　　Salary, Wages, and Related Expenses　　　　$2,368,000
　　Capital Expenditures　　　　　　　　　　　　495,000
　　Noncapital, Nonsalary Expenses　　　　　　　935,000
　　Investments　　　　　　　　　　　　　　　　100,000
　　Total Cash Outflows　　　　　　　　　　　$3,898,000

Ending Cash Balance　　　　　　　　　　　　　　-0-

ROLE OF THE PATIENT ACCOUNT MANAGER

The process of cash forecasting is probably one of the most important functions in hospital financial management. If properly used, the process can be the instrument that will help keep the hospital solvent because it will be able to predict cash shortfalls and take corrective actions such as:

- adjusting patient charges to meet expenses
- reducing expenses
- preparing for borrowings and/or investments

The patient account manager can play a vital role in this process. The following are some of the functions the patient account manager can and should perform:

Forecast Preparation:

1. Analyze patient accounts receivable by paying agent.
2. Identify the time lag factors for payments by paying agent.
3. Estimate the amount of bad debt writeoffs.
4. Calculate third party contractual allowances.
5. Estimate the amount of courtesy allowances and other similar deductions from gross patient charges.

Forecast Monitoring:

1. Assist in the preparation of the daily cash report (see Exhibit 10–1).
2. Maintain close communication between the patient business services department and the chief financial officer (CFO) and alert CFO to any potential trouble spots.

Exhibit 10–1 Daily Cash Report Form

```
               Memorial Hospital, Anytown, U.S.A.
                       Daily Cash Report
                   as of _____, 19 ___
```

	Today	Month-To-Date Actual	Budget
1. Beginning Cash Balance	$ _____	$ _____	$ _____
2. Plus:			
Cash Inflows:			
a. Net Return Accounts Receivable	$ _____	$ _____	$ _____
b. Other Operating Sources			
c. Borrowings			
d. Total Cash Inflows	$ _____	$ _____	$ _____
3. Total Cash On Hand (line 1 + line 2d)	$ _____	$ _____	$ _____
4. Less:			
Cash Outflows:			
a. Salary, Wages, and Related Expenses	$ _____	$ _____	$ _____
b. Capital Expenditures			
c. Noncapital, Nonsalary Expenses			
d. Investments			
e. Total Cash Outflows	$ _____	$ _____	$ _____
5. Ending Cash Balance (line 3 − line 4e)	$ _____	$ _____	$ _____

3. Maintain close communication with all major third party payers in order to expedite payments.
4. Maintain constant awareness of new systems and procedures which might expedite cash payments from all types of payers.

In summary, the patient account manager is responsible for the effective processing of the hospital's largest single asset—the patient accounts receivable. In this case, that means cash conversion—cash inflows. Because cash inflows are an integral part of the cash forecasting and management process, the patient account manager must be involved. If that is not the case, change is definitely indicated—the patient account manager had better become involved—to protect the hospital and his/her position as well.

NOTES

1. *Accreditation Manual for Hospitals* (Chicago: Joint Commission on Accreditation of Hospitals, 1981), p. 1.
2. Richard Baehr, *Cash Management* (Amherst, Mass.: Amherst Associates, Inc., 1979), pp. 79–82.
3. *Budgeting Manual*, 2nd ed. (Sacramento, Calif.: California Hospital Association, 1977), pp. 101–108.

Chapter 11

Analyzing the Financial Statements

Today, hospitals appear to be caught between two opposing forces:

- increased demand for more financial resources
- tightening of a very competitive money market

These conflicting forces make it absolutely vital for the hospital's financial management team to (1) keep abreast of developments in the external financial and legislative environment that may have an impact on the hospital's financial position, and (2) routinely analyze its internal financial position. By constantly analyzing and evaluating these factors, the hospital's financial management team can develop a cohesive financial plan that will assure the hospital's financial viability.

As a member of the hospital's financial management team, the patient account manager must assume an appropriate share of this responsibility. Consequently, the patient account manager must be thoroughly acquainted with techniques for analyzing financial statements, a process known as financial analysis. Financial analysis is a tool that can assist management in making rational decisions in keeping with the mission, goals, and objectives of the hospital. The purpose of this chapter is to acquaint the patient account manager with the more important ratios or tools used in financial analysis.

USE OF FINANCIAL RATIOS

To evaluate the financial condition and performance of a hospital, the financial management team needs a set of benchmarks or yardsticks. The benchmark most frequently used in financial analysis is known as either a ratio or an index. A ratio relates two segments of financial data, for example, gross patient accounts receivable and gross patient revenue, to each other. Analysis and interpretation of sets of ratios should give the experienced financial analyst a better understanding of the financial condition and performance of the hospital than he/she could obtain solely from the financial statements.

Financial analysis involves two types of comparisons. The first method of comparison involves evaluating performance of the hospital according to past, present, and forecasted ratio trends. When these ratios are displayed in a time series chart, as illustrated in Table 11-1, the analyst can study the changes and determine whether the financial condition and performance of the hospital has improved or deteriorated over a period of time. For easier interpretation, these data can be displayed in a graph similar to the one shown in Figure 11-1.

The second method of comparison involves comparing ratios of one hospital with those of another hospital, or with a regional, state, or national industry average (see Table 11-2). Again, for ease of interpretation, these data are displayed in the graph shown in Figure 11-2. In analyzing these data, it is important to avoid the assumption that industry averages represent the "gospel truth." On the other hand, the hospital that is substantially out of line with an industry average may well have a weakness in its financial performance. Therefore, substantial deviations from the averages should be investigated and corrective measures taken if necessary.

In many situations, it may be necessary to go well beyond reported figures and ratios to properly analyze the hospital's financial condition and performance. For example, Table 11-1 indicates that the percentage of gross patient accounts receivable to the gross patient revenue increased from

Table 11-1 Patient Accounts Receivable and Revenue: Five-Year Period

Memorial Hospital, Anytown, U.S.A.
Ratio Analysis of Gross Patient Accounts Receivable to Gross Patient Revenue
For the Five-Year Period Ending September 30, 19x5

Year	Gross Patient Revenue	Gross Patient Accounts Receivable	Ratio	Percent
19x1	$3,565,000	$582,400	6.1:1	16.3%
19x2	3,922,500	588,300	6.7:1	15.0
19x3	4,315,700	733,600	5.9:1	17.0
19x4	4,530,300	679,500	6.7:1	15.0
19x5	5,209,845	937,700	5.6:1	18.0

Analyzing the Financial Statements   221

Figure 11-1 Patient Accounts Receivable and Revenue: Five-Year Period

Memorial Hospital, Anytown, U.S.A.
Percent Ratio of Gross Patient Accounts Receivable to Gross Patient Revenue

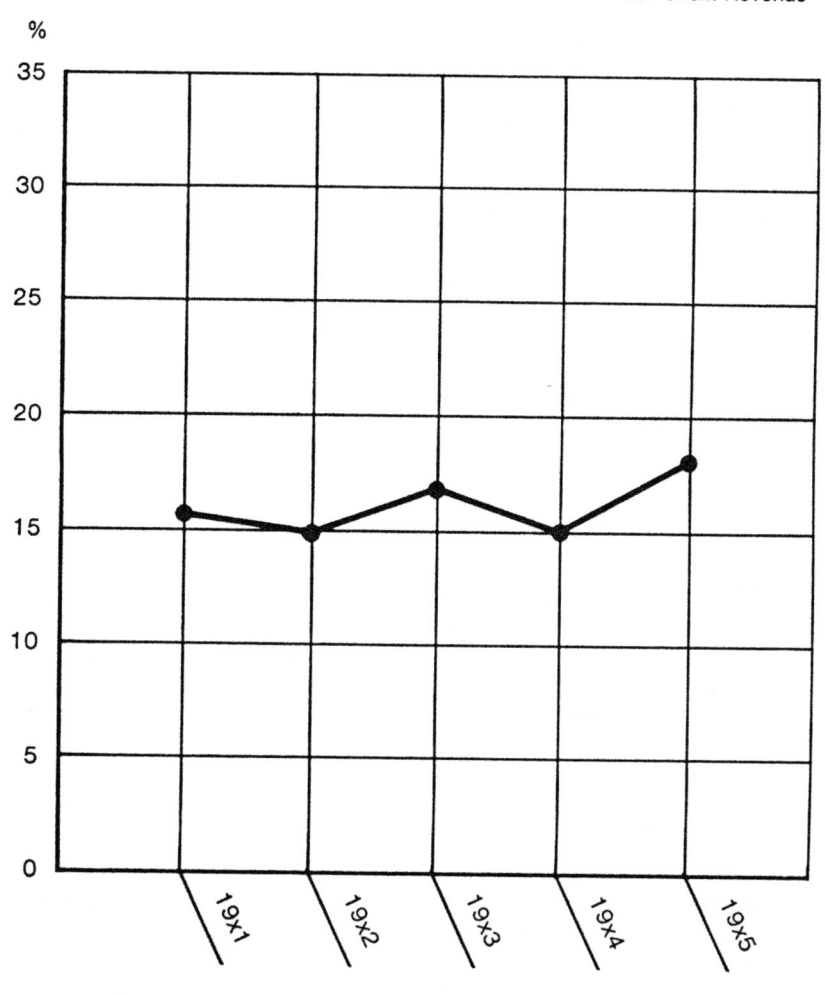

Year

Table 11-2 Comparative Analysis of Memorial Hospital to Regional Average of Percent of Gross Patient Accounts Receivable to Gross Patient Revenue

Year	Memorial Hospital	Regional Average	Variance Fav (Unfav)
19x1	16.3%	15.8%	(.5)%
19x2	15.0	15.4	.4
19x3	17.0	15.9	(1.1)
19x4	15.0	16.0	1.0
19x5	18.0	17.0	(1.0)

15.0 percent to 18.0 percent in years 19x4 and 19x5. Such a phenomenon could have any of the following causes:

- change in collection policy
- increase in rates
- slow pay by third party
- change in paying agent mix

These or many other reasons could have produced this adverse trend. Investigation and resolution of the problem is the responsibility of the patient account manager.

A word of caution about the use of industry standards is necessary here: it is important to compare apples to apples, not apples to oranges. Even with industry standards, the analyst must use discretion in interpreting the comparisons.

TYPES OF RATIO ANALYSIS

For the purposes of this discussion, financial ratios will be divided into five major categories:

1. liquidity
2. leverage
3. activity
4. profitability
5. profit planning

The first two kinds of ratios are developed from information on the statement of condition, or balance sheet. The three remaining types of ratios

Analyzing the Financial Statements 223

Figure 11-2 Comparative Analysis of Memorial Hospital to Regional Average of Percent of Gross Patient Accounts Receivable to Gross Patient Revenue

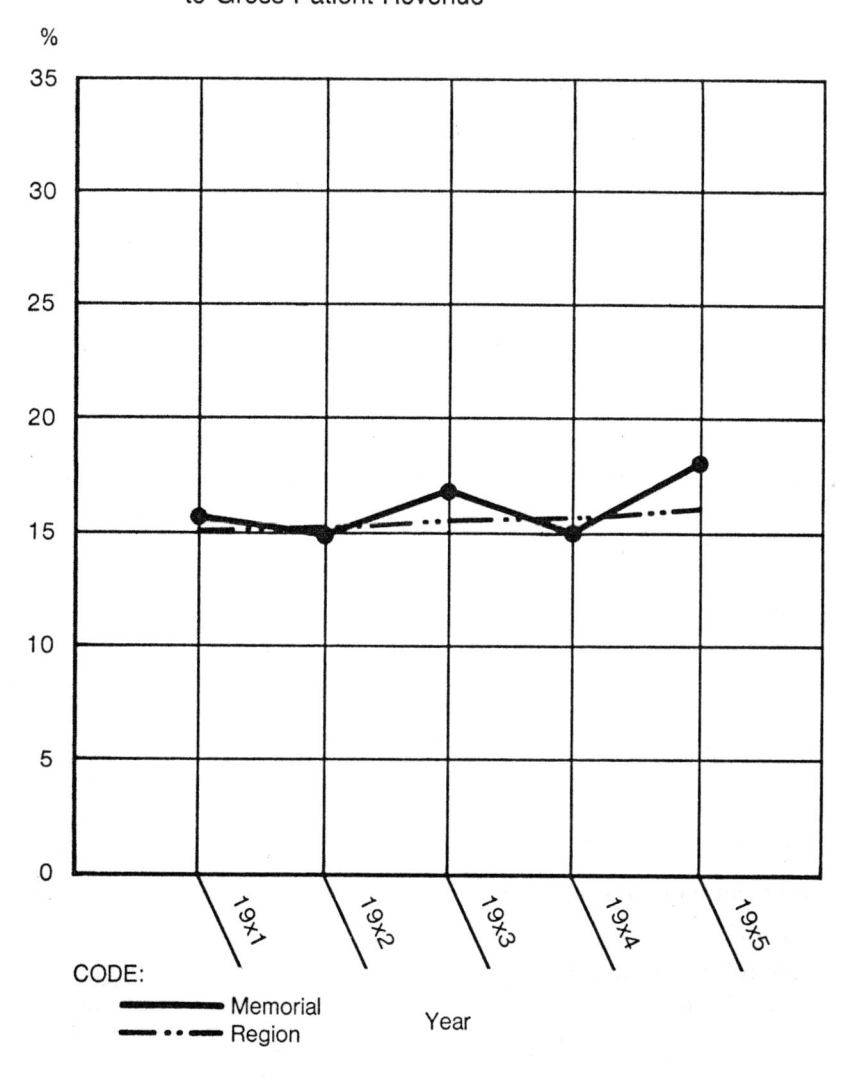

are based on information from the statement of operations, or the income statement, or from both statements. In analyzing the financial condition of a hospital, it is important to keep in mind that no single ratio or index will give the analyst the total picture. The analyst must therefore consider and evaluate a considerable number of ratios before drawing any final conclusion. Further, the analyst should not limit the analysis to just one year. It is preferable to consider three or more years to identify trends. For example, although the data for one year may indicate a rather weak financial position, it may actually reveal a favorable trend when compared to data for previous years.

Liquidity Ratios

Generally, the first concern of the hospital's financial analyst is the institution's liquidity. Liquidity ratios help to identify and evaluate the hospital's ability to meet its maturing short-term obligations. These ratios compare the hospital's current assets with its current liabilities. Current assets are assets normally and/or easily converted into cash within one year or less. Current liabilities, on the other hand, are debts due within one year or less.

The most commonly used liquidity ratio is the current ratio, which is computed by dividing current liabilities into current assets. Table 11–3, a statement of condition for Memorial Hospital, indicates that current assets for 19x2 include:

	Year 19x2
Operating cash	$ 45,000
Short-term investments	175,000
Net patient accounts receivable	1,310,000
Other receivables	170,000
Inventory	215,000
Prepaid expenses	85,000
Total current assets	$2,000,000

The current liabilities include:

Accounts payable	$ 285,000
Payroll taxes payable	350,000
Accrued payroll payable	420,000
Due to third party agencies	445,000
Total current liabilities	$1,500,000

The formula for the current ratio is:

$$\text{Current ratio} = \frac{\text{Current assets}}{\text{Current liabilities}}$$

or

$$1.33 = \frac{\$2,000,000}{\$1,500,000}$$

In this illustration, Memorial Hospital has 1.33 times as many current assets as current liabilities. Even though the current ratio is one of the generally accepted measures of liquidity or short-term solvency, its one weakness is the fact that it does not give adequate weight to the fact that $300,000 of the hospital's current assets are tied up in inventory and prepaid expenses that cannot be readily converted to cash.

The quick ratio, also known as the acid test ratio, can be used to compensate for this drawback in the current ratio. The quick ratio is computed by deducting inventories and prepaid expenses from current assets and dividing the balance by current liabilities. The quick ratio formula is:

$$\text{Quick ratio or acid test ratio} = \frac{\text{Current assets} - (\text{Inventory} + \text{Prepaid expenses})}{\text{Current liabilities}}$$

or

$$1.13 = \frac{\$1,700,000}{\$1,500,000}$$

The analyst will also see that $1,310,000 of the $1,700,000 remaining current assets is tied up in patient accounts receivable, and an additional $170,000 in other receivables. The following is a distribution analysis of the current assets, excluding inventories and prepaid expenses:

	Amount	Percent
Operating cash	$ 45,000	2.68
Short-term investments	150,000	8.96
Net patient accounts receivable	1,310,000	78.21
Other receivables	170,000	10.15
Net current assets	$1,675,000	100.00

Since the receivables represent such a significant share of the hospital's current assets, a special set of ratios will be presented later in this chapter.

Table 11–3 Comparative Statement of Condition

Memorial Hospital, Anytown, U.S.A.
Comparative Statement of Condition
As of September 30, 19x2

Assets	19x2		19x1		Change Increase (Decrease) Amount	Percent
Current Assets:						
Operating Cash		$ 45,000		$ 50,000	$ (5,000)	10.0%
Short-Term Investments		175,000		135,000	40,000	29.6
Gross Patient Accounts Receivable	$ 1,485,000		$ 1,363,000		122,000	9.0
Less: Reserves for Uncollectibles	175,000		160,000		15,000	9.4
Net Patient Accounts Receivable		$ 1,310,000		$1,203,000	107,000	8.9
Other Receivables		170,000		150,000	20,000	13.3
Inventory		215,000		195,000	20,000	10.3
Prepaid Expenses		85,000		72,000	13,000	18.1
Total Current Assets		$ 2,000,000		$1,805,000	195,000	10.8
Fixed Assets:						
Land		$ 50,000		$ 50,000	-0-	0.0
Plant and Equipment	$12,765,000		$11,320,000		$1,445,000	12.8
Less: Accumulated Depreciation	3,930,000		3,750,000		180,000	4.8
Net Plant and Equipment		$ 8,835,000		$7,570,000	$1,265,000	16.7
Total Fixed Assets		$ 8,885,000		$7,620,000	$1,265,000	16.7
Total Assets		$10,885,000		$9,425,000	$1,460,000	15.5

Analyzing the Financial Statements 227

Current Liabilities:			
Accounts Payable	$ 285,000	$ 260,000	9.6%
Payroll Taxes Payable	$ 350,000	$ 320,000	9.4
Accrued Payroll Payable	$ 420,000	$ 390,000	7.7
Short-term Note Payable	$ -0-	$ 60,000	100.0
Due to Third Party Agencies	$ 445,000	$ (60,000)	2.3
Total Current Liabilities	$ 1,500,000	$ 10,000	2.4
		$1,465,000	
Fixed Liabilities:			
Mortgage Payable	$ 5,790,000	$5,560,000	4.1
Total Fixed Liabilities	$ 5,790,000	$5,560,000	4.1
Total Liabilities	$ 7,290,000	$7,025,000	3.8
Net Worth:			
Beginning Balance	$ 2,400,000	$1,600,000	50.0
Plus: Operating Profit (Loss)	$ 1,195,000	$ 800,000	49.3
Ending Balance	$ 3,595,000	$2,400,000	49.8
Total Net Worth	$ 3,595,000	$2,400,000	49.8
Total Liabilities and Net Worth	$10,885,000	$9,425,000	15.5

Leverage Ratios

Leverage ratios, which measure the equity generated by the hospital compared with the financing provided by the hospital's creditors, have a number of implications. First, creditors look to the equity or owner-supplied funds to provide a margin of safety. If the owners provide only a small proportion of the total financing, the risks of the hospital are borne mainly by the creditors. Second, by raising funds through borrowing, the hospital gains the benefit of maintaining control with limited investment. Third, if the hospital earns more on the borrowed funds than it pays in interest, the return to the owners is increased. For example, if assets earn 14 percent and debt costs 12 percent, the 2 percent differential accrues to the hospital's benefit. Of course, leverage works both ways: if the return on assets falls to 10 percent, for example, the differential between that figure and the cost of debt must be covered by the hospital's equity or total profits. In the first instance, where assets earn more than debt costs, leverage is favorable; in the second, it is unfavorable.

Generally, leverage is evaluated two ways. The first method involves examining balance sheet ratios and determining the extent to which borrowed funds have been used to finance the hospital. The second approach measures the risks of debt with income statement ratios designed to determine the number of times fixed charges are covered by operating profits. These ratios are complementary, and most analysts use both kinds of leverage ratios.[1]

The debt ratio measures the percentage of total assets that has been provided by the hospital's creditors. Total debt includes current liabilities as well as long-term obligations. Creditors prefer moderate debt ratios, because the lower the ratio, the greater the protection for creditors against losses in the event of liquidation. The formula for the debt ratio is:

$$\text{Debt ratio} = \frac{\text{Total liabilities (debt)}}{\text{Total assets}}$$

or

$$66.97\% = \frac{\$7,290,000}{\$10,885,000}$$

In this case, Memorial Hospital has financed 66.97 percent of its assets through debt. This represents a substantial amount of debt. In all probability, prospective lenders would be reluctant to loan any more money to the hospital. If the hospital's debt ratio were 50 percent or less, it would be in a much better position to borrow additional money.

The times interest earned ratio measures the extent to which the hospital's profits can decline before it will lose the ability to meet its annual interest costs. Failure to meet interest expense could bring legal action from the hospital's creditors and possible bankruptcy.

Table 11–4, a statement of operations for Memorial Hospital, provides the profit and interest expense data necessary to compute the times interest earned ratio. The formula for the times interest earned ratio is:

$$\text{Times interest earned ratio} = \frac{\text{Profit before taxes + Interest expense}}{\text{Interest expense}}$$

or

$$= \frac{\$1,195,000 + \$492,150}{\$492,150}$$

or

$$3.43 \text{ times} = \frac{\$1,687,150}{\$492,150}$$

In this illustration, the hospital's gross income or profit available to service the $492,150 interest expense is $1,687,150, so the interest expense is covered only 3.43 times. If the industry average were 7.0 times, the hospital would be covering its interest expense with a minimal margin of safety; thus, it would be likely to have a low credit rating.

Fixed charges coverage analysis determines the number of times fixed charges are covered by the hospital's profit. Fixed charges include such items as interest, lease payments, rent, and sinking fund requirements. This ratio is more revealing than the times interest earned ratio because it includes other fixed costs that the hospital must meet to stay in business. The formula for fixed charge coverage is:

$$\text{Fixed charge coverage} = \frac{\text{Operating profit}}{\text{Interest + Rent + Leases + Other fixed charges}}$$

or

$$= \frac{\$1,195,000}{\$492,150 + \$205,000}$$

Table 11-4 Comparative Statement of Operations

Memorial Hospital, Anytown, U.S.A.
Comparative Statement of Operations
For Years Ending September 30, 19x2 and 19x1

	19x2 Amount	19x2 Percent	19x1 Amount	19x1 Percent	Change Amount	Change Percent
Volume						
Inpatient Days	28,567		28,564		12	0.1
Inpatient Admissions	3,402		3,173		229	7.1
Outpatient Visits	11,029		9,840		1,189	12.1
Revenue						
Gross Charges:						
Inpatient Services	$8,172,900	95.0	$7,309,620	95.5	$863,280	11.8
Outpatient Services	430,150	5.0	344,430	4.5	85,720	24.9
Gross Patient Charges	$8,603,050	100.0	$7,654,050	100.0	$949,000	12.4
Less: Provision for Bad Debts and Allowances	2,026,650	24.1	1,744,800	22.8	331,850	19.0
Net Patient Charges	$6,526,400	75.9	$5,909,250	77.2	$617,150	10.4
Other Operating Revenue	270,000	3.1	214,000	2.8	56,000	26.2
Total Revenue	$6,796,400	79.0	$6,123,250	80.0	$673,150	11.0
Expenses						
Administrative and Household	$ 924,250	* 10.8	$ 964,700	* 12.6	$ (40,450)	(4.2)
Employee Health and Welfare	481,720	5.6	431,180	5.6	50,540	11.7
General Professional Care	1,938,080	22.5	1,804,580	23.6	133,500	7.4
Auxiliary Services	1,327,530	* 15.4	1,229,670	* 16.0	97,860	8.0
Ambulatory Services	257,760	3.0	255,520	3.3	2,150	0.8
Depreciation	180,000	2.1	165,000	2.2	15,000	9.1
Interest Expense	492,150	5.7	472,600	6.2	19,550	4.1
Total Expenses	$5,601,400	65.1	$5,323,250	69.5	$278,150	5.2
Profit (Loss)	$1,195,000	13.9	$ 800,000	10.5	$395,000	49.3

or

$$1.7 \text{ times} = \frac{\$1,195,000}{\$697,150}$$

As was the case with the times interest earned ratio, the fixed charges coverage ratio is substantially low. If the industry average is 3.5 times, a potential lender would probably rate Memorial Hospital low as a credit risk.

Another ratio used to measure liquidity is one that helps to determine the hospital's defensive position. This ratio, known as the basic defensive interval, measures the interval of time the hospital can operate on its existing liquid assets without having to resort to cash flows from sales or other sources.[2] The basic defensive interval formula is:

$$\text{Basic defensive interval} = \frac{\text{Current assets} - \text{Inventory} - \text{Prepaid expenses}}{\text{Projected daily operating expenses} - \text{Depreciation}}$$

or

$$= \frac{\$2,000,000 - \$215,000 - \$85,000}{(\$5,601,400 - \$180,000) \div 365}$$

or

$$114.45 \text{ days} = \frac{\$1,700,000}{\$14,853}$$

Defensive assets include cash, investments, and net patient receivables. The denominator of the equation consists of projected net daily operating expenses of the hospital. It has been argued that this measure and other related measures give a more meaningful picture of liquidity than do the liquidity ratios considered so far.[3]

Activity Ratios

Activity ratios measure how efficiently the hospital is using its assets. Generally, the term "turnover rate" is used to show the number of times a particular asset is replenished in one year. This ratio is frequently used to measure the efficiency of handling of inventory and accounts receivable. One method used to compute the turnover rate for these two assets is:

$$\text{Inventory turnover to charges} = \frac{\text{Gross charges}}{\text{Inventory}}$$

or

$$40.01 \text{ times} = \frac{\$8,603,050}{\$215,000}$$

Another way to measure inventory turnover is:

$$\text{Inventory turnover to purchases} = \frac{\text{Purchases}}{\text{Inventory}}$$

Assume that during the year 19x2, Memorial Hospital purchased $1,935,000 worth of stock and supplies that were processed through its inventory system. The inventory turnover rate would be computed as follows:

$$9.00 \text{ times} = \frac{\$1,935,000}{\$215,000}$$

Generally, the more frequently an inventory turns over, the greater the efficiency. However, an inventory could have such a high turnover rate that the hospital is constantly out of stock and reorder costs could be substantially high; hence, a lower turnover rate might actually be more economical.

Fixed asset turnover is another ratio that is frequently used to evaluate the use of the hospital's fixed assets compared to its gross charges. The formula for the fixed asset turnover ratio is:

$$\frac{\text{Fixed assets turnover}}{\text{(gross charges)}} = \frac{\text{Gross charges to patients}}{\text{Fixed assets}}$$

or

$$0.97 \text{ times} = \frac{\$8,603,050}{\$8,885,000}$$

This formula can also be applied to the hospital's net charges to patients as follows:

$$\frac{\text{Fixed assets}}{\text{turnover (net)}} = \frac{\text{Net charges to patients}}{\text{Fixed assets}}$$

or

$$0.74 \text{ times} = \frac{\$6{,}526{,}400}{\$8{,}885{,}000}$$

The total asset turnover ratio compares the hospital's total assets to either the gross or net charges to patients as follows:

$$\frac{\text{Total asset}}{\text{turnover (gross)}} = \frac{\text{Gross charges to patients}}{\text{Total assets}}$$

or

$$0.79 \text{ times} = \frac{\$8{,}603{,}050}{\$10{,}885{,}000}$$

$$\frac{\text{Total asset}}{\text{turnover (net)}} = \frac{\text{Net charges to patients}}{\text{Total assets}}$$

or

$$0.60 \text{ times} = \frac{\$6{,}526{,}400}{\$10{,}885{,}000}$$

Accounts receivable turnover is another activity ratio that will be discussed in more detail later in this chapter.

Profitability Ratios

Profitability ratios measure the hospital's overall effectiveness in terms of generating profits compared with the hospital's revenue and investment. Since profitability ratios can be calculated for either gross or net charges to patients, the following examples will illustrate both types of ratios. When a hospital is required to pay income taxes, the net profit after taxes should always be used. The formulas are:

$$\text{Profit margin on gross charges} = \frac{\text{Net profit after taxes}}{\text{Gross charges to patients}}$$

or

$$13.89\% = \frac{\$1,195,000}{\$8,603,050}$$

$$\text{Profit margin on net charges} = \frac{\text{Net profit after taxes}}{\text{Net charges to patients}}$$

or

$$18.31\% = \frac{\$1,195,000}{\$6,526,400}$$

The profit margin ratio relates the net profit to either gross or net charges to patients. The resulting percentage indicates to management the degree of protection it has from falling charges or rising costs. The higher the percentage or margin, the less risk there is of losses due to reduced income or volume.

The return on total assets ratio compares the hospital's profit after taxes with its total assets. The formula for the ratio is:

$$\text{Return on total assets} = \frac{\text{Net profit after taxes}}{\text{Total assets}}$$

or

$$10.98\% = \frac{\$1,195,000}{\$10,885,000}$$

The return on net worth or equity ratio measures the net profit after taxes compared with the hospital's total net worth or owner's equity. The formula for this ratio is:

$$\text{Return on net worth (equity)} = \frac{\text{Net profit after taxes}}{\text{Net worth}}$$

or

$$33.24\% = \frac{\$1,195,000}{\$3,595,000}$$

This ratio gives management a benchmark for comparing what the hospital is earning with what it might obtain from another form of investment, for example, money market funds and new business.

Profit Planning Ratios

Break-even analysis ratios are used to determine profit for specific time periods, volumes, charges (net income), and patient mixes. Before a break-even analysis can be made, all the hospital's costs must be separated into fixed and variable costs. In addition, components known as contribution and the contribution margin are also incorporated into break-even analysis. Contribution is the dollar difference between the net charge or rate for a unit of service. The contribution margin is the difference, expressed as a percentage, between the net charge or rate. For example, assume that the average net charge (after provision for bad debts and allowances) for a one-day patient stay is $250. Assume further that the variable expense is $150. The computation of the contribution and the contribution margin would be as follows:

	Amount	Percent
Average daily net charge per patient day	$250.00	100.0%
Average variable cost per patient day	150.00	60.0%
Average contribution per patient day	$100.00	
Average contribution margin per patient day		40.0%

The break-even analysis identifies the point at which total revenue equals total expense plus the desired profit margin.

Using the data given above, assume that the hospital's average daily fixed costs are $15,000. Further assume that the hospital has targeted an average daily profit of $3,000. To accomplish these results, the hospital's daily break-even census would be:

Average daily net charge per patient day	$250.00
Average daily variable cost per patient day	$150.00
Average contribution per patient day	$100.00
Average daily fixed costs per patient day	$15,000
Target average daily net profit	$ 3,000
Average daily fixed costs and profit	$18,000
Break-even census ($18,000 ÷ $100)	180 patient days

The arithmetic method of computing the break-even point is one approach; another approach is to use formulas. The following formula can be used.

$$\frac{\text{Break-even point in}}{\text{units of service}} = \frac{\text{Fixed costs + Net profit}}{\text{Contribution}}$$

or

$$= \frac{\$15,000 + \$3,000}{\$100}$$

or

$$180 \text{ units} = \frac{\$18,000}{\$100}$$

If the analyst wants to compute the break-even net charges, the following formula could be used:

$$\frac{\text{Break-even point in}}{\text{dollars (net charges)}} = \frac{\$15,000 + \$3,000}{0.40}$$

or

$$\$45,000 = \frac{\$18,000}{0.40}$$

Another application of break-even analysis is determination of the margin of safety, that is, the percentage by which net charges can decline before the hospital experiences a loss. This percentage is a dramatic way of demonstrating to management how close the net charge level is to the break-even point (excluding profit).

Using the following data, the margin of safety can be computed as follows:

Total net charges	$45,000
Contribution margin	40%
Contribution	$18,000
Break-even charges (without profit)	$37,500
Profit	$ 3,000

$$\text{Margin of safety} = \frac{\text{Profit}}{\text{Contribution}}$$

or

$$16.67\% = \frac{\$3,000}{\$18,000}$$

and

$$\text{Margin of safety} = \frac{\text{Net charges} - \text{Break-even net charges}}{\text{Net charges}}$$

or

$$= \frac{\$45,000 - \$37,500}{\$45,000}$$

or

$$16.67\% = \frac{\$7,500}{\$45,000}$$

Thus, net charges of $45,000 could decline 16.67 percent (or $7,500) to $37,500 before the hospital would experience an operating loss.

To prove this analysis, the analyst can use the following procedure:

	Target Plan		Safety Test	
	Amount	Percent	Amount	Percent
Net Charges	$45,000	100.0%	$37,500	100.0%
Variable Expenses	27,000	60.0%	22,500	60.0%
Contribution	$18,000	40.0%	$15,000	40.0%
Fixed Costs	15,000		15,000	
Profit	$ 3,000		-0-	

LIQUIDITY OF PATIENT ACCOUNTS RECEIVABLE

Excluding fixed assets and equipment, the patient accounts receivable represent the hospital's largest single asset. To regard all receivables as liquid when in fact a sizable portion of them may be past due and/or uncollectible overstates the liquidity of the hospital. Receivables are liquid assets only to the extent that they can be collected within a reasonable amount of time. For this reason, it is imperative that the hospital establish an appropriate policy to take into account uncollectible accounts and contractual allowances. While patient accounts receivable may be analyzed as either gross or net, the most realistic approach is to base the analysis on net patient accounts receivable. However, in the following analysis of Memorial Hospital's patient accounts receivable, both methods will be used.

The most commonly used accounts receivable analysis is the number of days of average daily revenue uncollected or the average collection period ratio. This ratio is computed as follows:

	Gross Patient Accounts Receivable	Net Patient Accounts Receivable
1. Annual Charges to Patients	$8,603,050	$6,526,400
2. Number of Calendar Days	365	365
3. Average Daily Charges (line 1 ÷ line 2)	$ 23,570	$ 17,880
4. Patient Accounts Receivable	$1,485,000	$1,310,000
5. Average Collection Period (line 4 ÷ line 3)	63.0	73.3

Another ratio frequently used to analyze patient accounts receivable is the turnover rate. The following is the computation of Memorial Hospital's accounts receivable turnover rate:

	Gross Patient Accounts Receivable	Net Patient Accounts Receivable
1. Total Annual Patient Charges	$8,605,050	$6,526,400
2. Patient Accounts Receivable	$1,485,000	$1,310,000
3. Accounts Receivable Turnover Rate (line 1 ÷ line 2)	5.8 times	4.9 times

The cardinal rule in analyzing patient accounts receivable is to always compare gross charges to gross receivables and net charges to net receivables. Never compare gross charges to net receivables or vice versa.

Analyzing the Financial Statements   239

Another ratio used to analyze patient accounts receivable is the receivables to charges ratio. It is calculated as follows:

	Gross Patient Accounts Receivable	Net Patient Accounts Receivable
1. Patient Accounts Receivable	$1,485,000	$1,310,000
2. Annual Patient Charges	$8,603,050	$6,526,400
3. Receivables Percent of Charges (line 1 ÷ line 2)	17.26%	20.1%

While the above ratio compares the patient accounts receivable and patient account charges, the following analyses compare the receivables with both the hospital current and total assets as follows:

	Gross Patient Accounts Receivable	Net Patient Accounts Receivable
1. Patient Accounts Receivable	$1,485,000	$1,410,000
2. Current Assets	$2,000,000	$2,000,000
3. Percent of Current Assets (line 1 ÷ line 2)	74.3%	65.5%

	Gross Patient Accounts Receivable	Net Patient Accounts Receivable
1. Patient Accounts Receivable	$ 1,485,000	$1,310,000
2. Total Assets	$10,885,000	$9,425,000
3. Percent of Total Assets (line 1 ÷ line 2)	13.6%	13.9%

While the above analyses identify the percent of the hospital's assets tied up in patient accounts receivable, the following ratio computes the relationship of the hospital's net worth or equity to its patient accounts receivable:

	Gross Patient Accounts Receivable	Net Patient Accounts Receivable
1. Patient Accounts Receivable	$1,485,000	$1,310,000
2. Net Worth (equity)	$3,595,000	$3,595,000
3. Percent of Net Worth (line 1 ÷ line 2)	41.3%	36.4%

The ratio of patient accounts receivable to net worth could also be expressed as follows: (a) 1:2.4 (gross patient accounts receivable), and (b) 1:2.7 (net patient accounts receivable).

Finally the patient accounts receivable can be evaluated by computing the opportunity costs the hospital experiences by having its assets tied up in patient accounts receivable when they could be invested in a money market fund or other interest-bearing investment account. This opportunity cost is computed in the following manner:

	Gross Patient Accounts Receivable	Net Patient Accounts Receivable
1. Patient Accounts Receivable	$1,485,000	$1,310,000
2. Current Rate of Interest on Money Market Funds or Desired Rate of Return on Investment	15%	15%
3. Total Opportunity Costs per Year (line 1 × line 2)	$ 222,750	$ 196,500

If the average collection periods computed previously of 63.0 and 73.3 days were reduced by 10 days, the hospital's patient accounts receivable would be:

	Gross Patient Accounts Receivable	Net Patient Accounts Receivable
1. Patient Accounts Receivable	$1,485,000	$1,310,000
2. Average Daily Charges	$ 23,570	$ 17,880

	Gross Patient Accounts Receivable	Net Patient Accounts Receivable
3. Target Reduction of Number of Days	10	10
4. Amount to be Reduced (line 2 × line 3)	$ 235,700	$ 178,800
5. Current Rate of Interest on Money Market Funds	15%	15%
6. Opportunity Savings per Year (line 4 × line 5)	$ 35,355	$ 26,820

In this illustration, Memorial Hospital gains a one-time increase in working capital of $235,700 (gross) or $178,880 (net), as well as the opportunity to earn $35,355 (gross) or $26,832 (net) by investing in a money market fund.

ANOTHER LOOK AT FINANCIAL STATEMENTS

The statement of condition in Table 11-3, pages 226-227, illustrated the necessity of having financial data for more than one year. If the analyst only has data for one year, there is absolutely no basis for evaluating changes. The illustrated statement displays results for two years side by side, and identifies the dollar and percent change from the first year to the second. These changes are summarized in the statement of changes in financial position in Table 11-5.

The statement of changes in financial position identifies the specific changes, uses, and sources of working capital, as well as how the hospital's income was provided and how it was applied. The reader should keep the following formula in mind as a method of showing the source of funds:

- Cash flow = Net operating profits + Depreciation.

Net operating profit plus any noncash expenses such as depreciation is the only source of funds, other than borrowing of some kind. Of course, the hospital cannot maintain its viability and grow without profit.

The statement of operations in Table 11-4 is also based on two years' data. In studying the illustration, note that each year's dollar operating results are analyzed as a percentage of the hospital's gross patient charges. This type of analysis allows the analyst to compare the change in either revenue or expense mix. For example, outpatient revenue increased as a

Table 11–5 Statement of Changes in Financial Position

Memorial Hospital, Anytown, U.S.A.
Statement of Changes in Financial Position
From September 30, 19x1 to September 30, 19x2

Funds Provided By:		
Net Operating Profit	$1,195,000	
Depreciation	180,000	
Total Funds Provided from Operations	$1,375,000	
Funds Applied To:		
Purchase of Plant and Equipment	$1,445,000	
Increase of Mortgage Payable	(230,000)	
Increase in Working Capital (see below)	160,000	
Total Funds Applied from Operations	$1,375,000	

Changes in Working Capital

Uses:		
Decrease in Operating Cash	$ (5,000)	
Increase in Short-term Investments	40,000	
Increase in Net Accounts Receivable	107,000	
Increase in Other Receivables	20,000	
Increase in Inventory	20,000	
Increase in Prepaid Expenses	$13,000	
Net Uses of Working Capital		$195,000
Sources:		
Increase in Accounts Payable	$ 25,000	
Increase in Payroll Payable	30,000	
Increase in Accrued Payroll Payable	30,000	
Decrease in Short-term Note Payable	(60,000)	
Increase in Amount Due to Third Party	10,000	
Net Sources of Working Capital		$ 35,000
Net Increase in Working Capital		$160,000

percentage of gross patient charges from 4.5% in 19x1 to 5.0% in 19x2, and administrative and household expenses declined from 12.6% in 19x1 to 10.8% in 19x2. As in the statement of condition, the statement of operations shows changes in both dollars and percentages.

To summarize, in analyzing financial statements some basis for comparing current data is essential. The following information represents some of the bases that can be used for comparing current operating results:

- budget or financial plan
- actual results for the previous month or year
- national, regional, or special industry indexes

The important issue to keep in mind is that a single accounting period's financial or production results are virtually meaningless unless they can be compared to something. The types of financial analyses, ratios, and statements that can be used for such comparisons are limited only by the analyst's imagination. Regardless of what methods are used, intelligent comparisons and analyses that lead to appropriate management decisions and corrective action are vital to the future of the hospital.

NOTES

1. J. Fred Weston and Eugene F. Brigham, *Essentials of Managerial Finance* (New York: Holt, Rinehart and Winston, Inc., 1971), p. 43.
2. James C. Van Horne, *Financial Management and Policy* (Englewood Cliffs, N.J.: Prentice-Hall, Inc., 1971), p. 645.
3. Ibid.

Chapter 12

Payment and Collection for Services Rendered

In his book, *Managing in Turbulent Times,* Peter Drucker observes that hospitals must consider the cost of staying in business to be part of their operating costs. The problem, as Drucker sees it, is that hospitals treat any surplus of operating revenues over operating expenses as a profit that they are not supposed to make. As a result, they not only conceal their true costs, but also endanger their own future and impose burdens on society and on the wealth-producing capacity of the economy.[1]

No one can quarrel with Drucker's contention that profit is necessary to assure a hospital's continuing existence. Moreover, one can take this line of reasoning a step further and say that a hospital cannot survive unless that profit and its other related financial requirements are collected in cold hard cash.

No business can survive if all its revenues are tied up in accounts receivable, with only a small trickle of cash flowing in. It is the patient account manager's responsibility to assure that there is a constant and adequate flow of cash into the hospital and that there is an appropriate turnover rate for patient accounts receivable. Rate setting in relation to revenue was discussed in Chapter 9 of this book. This chapter will discuss payment systems. Basically, payment boils down to the total amount of cash the hospital actually receives for its services.

When one surveys the hospital industry, it is interesting to note that the payment system employed by the major purchasers of hospital care has dictated the type of system used to deliver that care at any particular time. For example, the forerunners of modern health insurance plans generally covered a specific number of days of hospitalization, for example, 21 days in a semi-private room, as well as the use of the operating room, laboratory service, drugs and dressings.[2] The number of subscribers was limited, and the emphasis was on hospitalization. The majority of patients was either self-pay or covered by some form of public assistance. The net effect was more bad debts but fewer contractual allowances.

After World War II, health insurance was improved, and coverage of major medical expenses evolved in response to sharply escalating health care costs. This coverage also paid for services such as ambulatory care, prescription drugs, and dentistry.[3] Nevertheless, the major emphasis continued to be on hospitalization, with relatively minimal coverage for ambulatory or clinical services. As a result, hospitals did little to encourage the development of ambulatory and related kinds of services. In this setting, the patient who had little or no coverage presented a cash flow problem for the hospital. To some extent, the problem was compensated for by the fact that the proportion of patients with commercial health insurance was steadily increasing, as is indicated in Table 12–1. Even after the advent of Medicare and Medicaid in 1966, the main emphasis of health insurers was still on hospitalization. As a result, there was still no incentive for the hospital industry to develop ambulatory and clinical services. Cash collection for inpatient services was easier than it was for outpatient services.

The growth in health insurance coverage assisted hospitals in collecting cash for services rendered because the formerly self-pay patient now had a third party guaranteeing payment for his/her care. The increase in third party coverage has helped make the job of the patient account manager a little easier because insurers pay the majority of a patient's inpatient bill.

Table 12–1 Number of Individuals Covered for Hospital Expenses (in millions)

Year	All Health Insurers	Commercial Insurers Total	Group Policies	Individual and Family Policies
1940	12.3	3.7	2.5	1.2
1945	32.1	10.5	7.8	2.7
1950	76.6	37.0	22.3	17.3
1955	105.5	57.3	39.0	24.1
1960	130.0	76.7	55.2	30.2
1965	148.8	87.0	66.5	36.1
1970	172.8	101.0	82.0	42.0
1971	175.8	104.1	82.1	45.0
1972	178.4	106.7	83.0	48.0
1973	182.1	108.7	83.5	50.9

Source: Jeffrey A. Prussin and Jack C. Wood, eds., "Private Third Party Reimbursement," *Topics in Health Care Financing* 2, no. 1 (Fall 1975): 5.

On the other hand, some third parties, that is, Medicare and Medicaid, which now dominate a major portion of the hospital market, dictate how much cash they will pay the hospital for services rendered to their subscribers.

In the late 1970s and early 1980s, both insurance companies and government third party payment agencies have increased their outpatient and preventive medicine benefits. Hospitals have reacted by changing their delivery systems. Same-day surgery centers, community health care centers, outpatient satellite clinics, and ambulatory care centers are now becoming much more common. To cope with all these changes, as well as to meet increased demands for cash, the patient account manager must adjust the operations of the hospital's patient business services department.

PUBLISHED CHARGE VERSUS PAYMENT

As stated earlier, one must distinguish between published charges and payment or reimbursement for services. Most hospitals have a catalog of all the services they provide, with a published charge for each of these services. As stated in Chapter 9, the published charge reflects the amount necessary to cover such financial requirements as:

- labor and related costs
- supplies and purchased services
- capital assets
- education and research
- bad debts and allowances
- profit and provision for growth

Regardless of the type of coverage, every patient who enters a given hospital is charged the same rate for the same service. Actual payment for services, however, is a different matter. The amount of cash the hospital actually receives depends on the type of coverage the patient has. With this in mind, the key point for the patient account manager to remember is that he/she must:

- maximize cash inflow
- minimize allowances

This can be accomplished in a number of ways. As an example, high risk patients can be placed in less costly, or lower charge, rooms.

CLASSIFICATION OF PAYERS

Generally, hospital patients can be divided into two major categories in terms of who pays for their care:

1. self-pay
2. third party

The self-pay patient either has no insurance coverage, is totally responsible for payment of his/her hospital bill, or must pay the balance of the cost of his/her care after the third party has paid its share. A third party payer can be an individual, an agency, an insurance company, or some type of prepaid plan that is obligated to pay all or part of a patient's hospital bill. Payment systems used by third party payers are usually based on the hospital's costs, charges, or a combination of the two. Some Blue Cross plans and most commercial insurance companies pay the hospital either full charges or a percentage of full charges, and the patient is responsible for the balance. Other Blue Cross plans, Medicare, and Medicaid pay the hospital according to individualized formulas based on a hospital's costs, "reasonable costs," or "allowable costs." There is also frequently either a deductible and/or a coinsurance portion that the patient must pay. Usually, there is a contractual allowance (the difference between the published charge and net cash received) for which the hospital has no recourse to the patient. Thus, the hospital must absorb the difference.

Through proper admitting and discharge procedures, the patient account manager can maximize cash inflow and minimize contractual allowances. The key is to learn the rules of the game and play it with imagination and integrity.

PAYMENT SYSTEMS

Basically, there are two payment systems in the hospital industry: (1) prospective, and (2) retrospective. Under prospective payment, the hospital and the purchaser of services determine in advance the amount the hospital will charge the purchaser for a specified period of time. A substantial number of Blue Cross plans and state agencies pay hospitals under prospective payment systems.[4]

Until 1972, when the Social Security Amendments in Public Law 92-603 were enacted, the virtually universal retrospective payment systems, that is, reimbursement, represented what amounted to a blank check for hospitals. The original retrospective reimbursement system allowed hospitals to spend money to provide services for third party subscribers. After the fiscal year ended and these expenditures were audited, the total costs were computed for each third party. If the hospital had spent more than it had been paid by the third party in the interim, the third party gave the hospital additional money. If final costs were less than these interim payments, the hospital returned the difference to the third party. For example, assume that Memorial Hospital's total costs were $3,000,000, and one-third of its patient days were covered by a cost-based third party. The third party's share of the total costs would be $1,000,000. Assume further that the third party has made interim payments totaling $1,050,000 to Memorial Hospital. The hospital would be required to return $50,000 to the third party. If, on the other hand, the hospital had received only $900,000 in interim payments, the third party would have to pay the hospital an additional $100,000.

Under this system, many hospitals were being paid for underutilization. They paid very little attention to the relationship of their charges and their costs. By introducing payment based on the lesser of charges or costs, Public Law 92-603 changed that. The payment of the lesser of costs or charges requires a hospital to keep its total charges above the third party's share of reimbursable costs. Otherwise, it will be paid only charges. For example, in the case cited above, if Memorial Hospital's total charges to the third party were $975,000, compared to its share of the costs, which was $1,000,000, the hospital would receive only $975,000. If, on the other hand, the charges were $1,100,000, the hospital would be reimbursed for cost, that is, $1,000,000.

SEGMENTATION OF PATIENT ACCOUNTS RECEIVABLE

Market segmentation is a common technique of market analysis. It identifies relevant characteristics of a population to be served and divides them into groups and subgroups. The demands and needs of each group are identified, and advertising and marketing campaigns that appeal to those specific needs are designed. The patient account manager can apply this technique to the management of patient accounts receivable through the use of a matrix or grid. This will enable him/her to maximize cash inflow and minimize contractual allowances.

The first step in segmenting patient accounts receivable is to divide the total account file into a minimum of six major classifications:

1. unbilled inhouse accounts
2. unbilled discharged inpatient accounts
3. unbilled outpatient accounts
4. billed inhouse accounts
5. billed discharged inpatient accounts
6. billed outpatient accounts

The account file should also be divided according to primary or major third party paying agent:

- self-pay
- Medicare
- Medicaid
- Blue Cross
- commercial insurance
- workmen's compensation

If one third party, a specific commercial insurance carrier, for example, accounts for a significant portion of the hospital's accounts, a separate classification should be created for that third party.

The classifications can then be arranged on a matrix similar to the one illustrated in Exhibit 12-1. Note that the matrix shows both the dollar amount and the percentage represented by each segment of the patient accounts receivable. This facilitates trend analysis and other studies of payment patterns.

Because each segment has unique billing and payment characteristics, the segmentation matrix helps the patient account manager isolate potential trouble spots and take corrective action.

The number of days of revenue uncollected is a key indicator in the analysis of each accounts receivable segment because each paying agent is likely to have a different hospital service utilization profile.

In summary, the segmentation matrix is another tool the patient account manager can use to expedite collection of cash. This technique, along with improvements that suit the needs of the individual hospital, should be incorporated into every hospital's management information system. The patient account manager must overcome any resistance to building the technique into the management information system by steadfastly maintaining that data processing is limited only by the imagination and ability of its designers and users. The patient account manager cannot perform effectively without adequate, accurate, and timely information, and segmentation analysis is an important part of that information. In the end, no one in the hospital gets paid if cash is not brought in; cash is the hospital's lifeblood.

MONITORING ACCOUNTS IN COLLECTION

Whether the hospital has an inhouse or outside collection agency, or uses both, appropriate devices for monitoring their relative effectiveness

Payment and Collection for Services 251

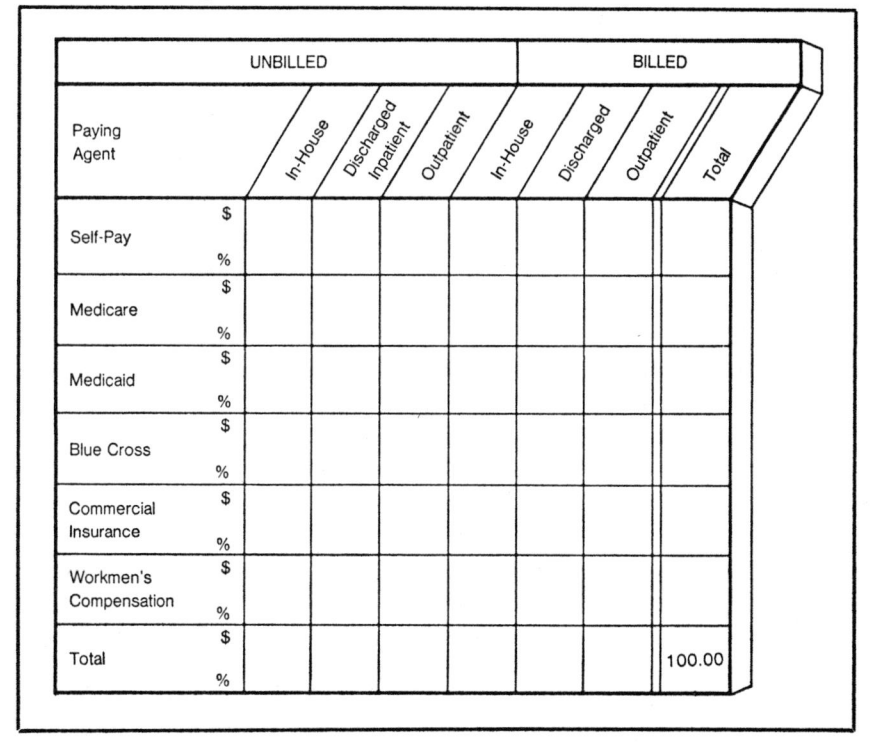

Exhibit 12-1 Segmentation Matrix of Patient Accounts Receivable

Paying Agent	UNBILLED			BILLED			
	In-House	Discharged Inpatient	Outpatient	In-House	Discharged	Outpatient	Total
Self-Pay $ %							
Medicare $ %							
Medicaid $ %							
Blue Cross $ %							
Commercial Insurance $ %							
Workmen's Compensation $ %							
Total $ %							100.00

and cost/benefit must be developed. The monitoring process should also serve as an internal audit system that protects the hospital from improper handling of accounts placed for collection.

The ten guidelines given below are essential for monitoring accounts referred to collection agencies:

1. Do have a written, board-approved policy for identifying and processing accounts classified as bad debts and uncollectibles.
2. Do have at least two individuals above the patient account manager—with one of them preferably a board member—responsible for reviewing and approving all referrals of accounts to collection agencies and all identification of accounts as uncollectible.
3. Do have at least two bonded collection agencies handle bad debt accounts, and have still another agency handle all accounts returned as uncollectible. (This measure is a final test of an account's actual uncollectibility.)
4. Do have a written agreement with every collection agency used that

stipulates that all accounts without payment activity within six months are to be returned to the hospital.
5. Do require the collection agency to obtain the hospital's approval in writing for any compromise settlements.
6. Do require that the hospital's internal or external auditors perform interim audits of the accounts referred to each collection agency.
7. Do require each collection agency to submit a monthly aged trial balance and progress reports on all accounts handled.
8. Do require the agency to have the hospital's written approval before undertaking litigation.
9. Do analyze and compare the collection effectiveness and net cost of each agency at least semiannually.
10. Do establish a balance sheet reserve account for all accounts referred to collection agencies. The method for establishing such an account is described below.

Reserve for Bad Debts

All patient accounts receivable should be reviewed monthly to determine their collectibility. Any account, regardless of age or length of time since discharge, considered to be a collection problem by the patient account manager should be identified and written off as a bad debt. The hospital accounting department will use the following compound journal entry to record accounts identified as bad debts and approved for collection.

Assume that Memorial Hospital bad debt accounts total $20,000:

Bad Debt Expense $20,000
Agency Accounts Receivable $20,000
   Reserve for Bad Debts $20,000
   Active Accounts Receivable $20,000

The debit entries record the amount to be written off as a bad debt expense in the statement of operations and establish an asset account in the statement of condition. The credit entries establish a reserve account to totally offset the agency accounts receivable asset account and remove the accounts from the active accounts receivable in the statement of condition.

To further illustrate these entries, assume that $500 is collected in cash. The following compound journal entry must be made:

Cash $500
Reserve for Bad Debts $500
   Recoveries from Bad Debts $500
   Agency Accounts Receivable $500

The debit entries increase the cash account and reduce the reserve account in the statement of condition. The credit entries reduce the bad debt expense on the statement of condition as well as the amount of agency accounts receivable.

To continue the illustration, if accounts totaling $5,000 were returned to the hospital as uncollectible, the following adjusting entry removes the accounts from the statement of condition:

Reserve for Bad Debts $5,000
 Agency Accounts Receivable.. $5,000

A permanent file should be established for accounts removed from the hospital's books because they are considered uncollectible. This file will serve as a collection record that the patient business services department staff can check when admitting patients. The check will reveal, among other facts, whether a patient being admitted has been a collection problem for the hospital in the past.

The ten guidelines and the system for handling bad debts and uncollectible accounts have these advantages:

- They provide control over bad debt accounts and ensure additional collection efforts after the hospital has exhausted its own.
- They provide for a realistic reserve for bad debts that can be adjusted and controlled monthly.
- They comprise a systematic means of exerting constant and ongoing vigilance over bad debt offenders.
- They enhance the hospital's ability to identify bad debts in advance.
- They improve the cash inflow from patient accounts receivable.

The systems and procedures described for monitoring and controlling accounts receivable are not ends in themselves. They should be considered a nucleus the hospital can use for evaluating and improving its present system. The hospital should analyze its system at least annually and make any adjustments dictated by changes in its socioeconomic environment.

OTHER METHODS OF IMPROVING PAYMENT

The hospital's socioeconomic environment changes constantly. Continual analysis and adjustment of accounts receivable management systems to adapt to these changes is one of the patient account manager's greatest responsibilities. The patient account manager's ultimate objective is to maximize cash inflow and minimize allowances. The bottom line is the amount of cash collected, not necessarily the amount of profit generated. Accordingly, hospital policies should be constantly reviewed and analyzed along with systems and procedures. These reviews and the resulting recommendations to the hospital board are a major responsibility of the patient account manager.

The first step in improving the hospital's cash inflow is to consider the cost of carrying patient accounts receivable. Opportunity costs were discussed earlier in this book; these costs are the cost to the hospital of carrying accounts receivable. Any hospital that does not charge interest on outstanding patient accounts is not only jeopardizing its own financial stability, but it is also imposing an additional burden on patients and third parties who do pay. Interest charges not only provide additional revenue but they also motivate debtors to pay hospital bills just as they pay utility, credit card, and other bills that impose finance charges. The hospital's true purpose is to provide health care; it should not be forced to act as a lending or financing institution.

Many hospitals require deposits from patients when they are admitted as inpatients or outpatients. The word "deposit" implies that all or part of the amount paid will be returned to the payer. This is far from reality. The word is misleading and does not convey the hospital's true intent, which is to get a "prepayment" for service. This point may seem petty, but hospitals must communicate with patients in a businesslike manner if they want to enhance payment for services.

The patient account manager can also enhance cash inflow by striving to reduce or eliminate lost charges and no charges. Medical charts should be routinely reviewed and compared with patient charges as part of the hospital's internal auditing process to ensure that all services that are rendered are charged for. Experience has proven that this type of internal audit and control will more than pay for the expense involved in conducting the audits.

In summary, the patient account manager must be constantly on the alert for any weaknesses within the hospital's systems and procedures. He/she must use the most valuable management tool of all—imagination—to maximize the hospital's cash inflow and minimize its allowances.

NOTES

1. Peter F. Drucker, *Managing in Turbulent Times* (New York: Harper & Row, 1980), p. 34.
2. Jeffrey A. Prussin and Jack C. Wood, eds., "Private Third Party Reimbursement," *Topics in Health Care Financing* 2, no. 1 (Fall 1975): 3.
3. Ibid., p. 3.
4. William L. Dowling, ed., "Prospective Rate Setting," *Topics in Health Care Financing* 3, no. 2 (Winter 1976): 1.

Chapter 13

Internal Audit and Control of Receivables

Until recently, many of the management tools generally accepted in industry were considered impractical for the hospital industry. Today, however, budgeting, cost accounting, productivity measurement, performance evaluation, and strategic planning are all examples of management tools that are enthusiastically embraced by hospital managers as vital tools in their efforts to operate more effectively and efficiently.

As hospitals have become larger and more complex, the gap between the administrative-financial departments and the professional services departments has widened. This phenomenon has required great changes in the managerial and technological tools employed by the hospital management team. On-line, realtime data processing systems, operations research, management by objectives, management engineering, simulation analysis, and marketing are just a few of the new concepts hospitals are using to increase productivity and profitability.

Each of these tools depends on financial and statistical data. The integrity of these data must be unquestionable. Therefore, built-in controls and audits must be developed and implemented to guarantee the accuracy and validity of the data.

Modern hospital management requires timely and accurate reports in order to properly analyze and control the activities for which it is responsible. The timeliness of these reports depends on the sophistication and efficiency of the system used to process the data. The accuracy of the reports depends on people and the extent to which they adhere to established procedures. The human element reminds us of Alexander Pope's classic observation that to err is human.[1] Internal audit and control can be used by the patient account manager to ensure the integrity of his/her management information.

INTERNAL AUDIT

An internal audit has been defined as an "independent appraisal of activity within an organization for the review of accounting, financial and other operations as a basis for service to management—a managerial control which functions by measuring and evaluating the effectiveness of other controls."[2] This definition is supplemented by a description of activities appropriate to the scope of an internal audit function. These activities include:[3]

- reviewing and appraising the soundness, adequacy and application of accounting, financial, and operating controls
- ascertaining the extent of compliance with established policies, plans, and procedures
- ascertaining the extent to which company assets are accounted for, and safeguarded from losses of all kinds
- ascertaining the reliability of accounting and other data developed within the organization
- appraising the quality of performance in carrying out assigned responsibilities

A key element of internal audit is the element of surprise. The very existence of an internal auditor and the realization that all activities within the organization are subject to scrutiny by an independent party encourages accuracy and compliance with established procedures.

The location of the internal auditor's position in the organizational chart depends on several factors, including:[4]

- site of the hospital
- method of accounting
- scope and depth of the internal audit program
- intensity or frequency of internal audits

Usually, the internal auditor reports to the chairman of the governing body or his/her designate. This reporting pattern gives the internal audit staff considerable independence from those whose work they audit. Independence of the internal audit function is further enhanced by correlating it with the audit work of the hospital's external auditor. In the resulting integrated audit program, the work of the internal auditor and the external auditor complements that of the other. An integrated audit program becomes even more important as the hospital's work volume grows, as the scope of the audit program is expanded, and as sophisticated technology is increasingly used.

INTERNAL CONTROL

Internal control is a management tool that can assist the hospital management team by building automatic devices into the management information system to ensure compliance with established policies, systems, and procedures. The internal control program also aids management in keeping policies and procedures current and in documenting all changes in them.

To achieve effective internal control, a hospital should:[5]

- establish an effective organization through which responsibility and authority can be delegated and exercised
- develop policies and procedures, consistent with the objectives and needs of the institution, to safeguard its assets, ensure the accuracy and reliability of accounting data, and promote operational efficiency and adherence to established policies

The American Institute of Certified Public Accountants defines internal control as a plan of organization and the coordinate methods and measures adopted within a business to safeguard its assets, *check* the accuracy and reliability of its accounting data, promote operational efficiency and encourage adherence to prescribed managerial policies.[6]

Kampmann states that, in its broadest meaning, internal control concerns all elements of management. Organization, staffing, planning, directing, and controlling are all cited directly or indirectly in the process. He also contends that it is doubtful that many accountants or financial managers think of internal control in such broad terms. Their tendency has been to view it more in terms of accounting controls, which are really only part of internal control.[7]

An effective internal control system has four fundamental elements:

1. *Separation of duties.* No one individual or department should account for its own activities or report on the results of its own operations. Stated simply, no one function should be contained or controlled by one individual.
2. *Organizational structure.* Responsibility and accountability must be well documented and defined through the use of an organizational chart and job descriptions that include specific measurements or expectations of acceptable performance.

3. *Sound policies and procedures.* The hospital's goals and objectives must be well defined, and corresponding policies must be established, documented, and communicated by the hospital's board to those employees who are responsible for carrying them out.
4. *Adequate staff of trained personnel.* The hospital must retain only employees who are well trained and knowledgeable about current practice in their profession or trade to ensure proper administration of the hospital's operations. An effective inservice education program for *all* employees can help ensure an enlightened and knowledgeable staff. The objective should be a competent, reliable, and stable staff capable of quality work and high productivity.

To summarize, internal audit and internal control are management tools that are primarily concerned with people. These tools are concerned with how well employees:

- follow prescribed procedures
- organize themselves for control purposes
- develop themselves professionally

It is imperative that *all* employees periodically review their objectives and take steps to ensure that internal controls implemented by the hospital management do indeed promote operational efficiency within the framework of the hospital's goals and objectives.[8]

FINANCIAL VERSUS OPERATIONAL AUDITING

The financial audit tests the integrity of the hospital's accounting and statistical records. Through a planned process that includes a variety of sampling, verification, and testing techniques, the internal and/or the external auditor can evaluate the creditability of the records. With the auditor's assurance of creditability of the records, management can make decisions with confidence that the data base it uses is sound.

While the financial audit concerns itself primarily with financial data, the operational audit concentrates on systems in an effort to spot weaknesses. As a representative of management, the operational auditor investigates activities to determine whether departments have a clear understanding of hospital and departmental objectives. The operational audit is also intended to verify whether departments:[9]

- properly maintain records
- accurately record information

- appropriately protect and manage cash, inventories, equipment, supplies, and personnel
- effectively interact with other departments

As is the case with the financial audit, the operational audit requires a detailed audit plan. This plan should provide for:

- planning and budgeting
- management information
- purchasing and storage
- equipment procurement and management
- management of facilities with an eye toward health and safety
- staffing
- performance standards

The operational audit ensures the effectiveness of the hospital's operational systems, as well as their conformity to management goals and objectives.[10]

EXTERNAL VERSUS INTERNAL AUDITING

Accuracy is the primary concern of both the external auditor and the internal auditor. The internal auditor conducts ongoing testing and evaluation of systems, procedures, and records; the external auditor provides the public and the governing board with an annual statement of opinion on the validity of the statements for the fiscal year. In addition, the external independent public auditor:

- appraises internal control systems
- compares effectiveness and operations of the hospital with those of similar institutions

One of the most valuable services the external auditor performs for the hospital is the management letter, which outlines any major weaknesses discovered during the audit process. Generally, the external audit and the internal audit processes are integrated into a set of complementary procedures that are effective, continuous devices for testing the accuracy of the hospital's records and systems at reasonable cost and with minimal duplication of effort.

All accounting and operating systems and subsystems have three basic control points: (1) entry; (2) processing; and (3) exit. The fundamental principle of internal control is the separation or segregation of duties. This means that no one individual is allowed to have complete control over all three basic control points.

Accounting information requires that precontrolled methods be used to ensure that every transaction is properly recorded. Prenumbered cash receipts and prenumbered checks are the simplest examples of such methods. They are intended to make certain that all transactions are recorded and in proper order.[11]

An example of entry point control is the midnight census. Hospitals have a fixed bed capacity that is not normally exceeded. Therefore, the number of inhouse patients and the revenue they represent, for accounting purposes, cannot be greater than the number recorded in the census report. To put it another way, a financial record must be established and revenue recorded for every patient listed on the census report.

The vital point to remember about entry point control is that all entry point data must be documented through cash register tapes, admitting logs, and so forth. These data comprise evidence for internal and external audits.

The key to processing point control is to monitor the recording and summarizing of accounting transactions to make sure they are complete and in balance. For example, the amount recorded in the general ledger as revenue from patients should match the total of the amounts of revenue posted to individual patient financial records.[12]

Exit point control requires extensive review of the results of accounting transactions to determine whether they have been appropriately documented. For example, a patient's medical record should contain:

- doctor's request for hospital services
- nurse's report of rendering services
- medical reports of rendering of ancillary department services

Each of these modes of service should be recorded and charged to the patient's financial record as they are performed.

Other examples of exit point control are financial ratios and predetermined performance standards, for example, number of days of average daily revenue uncollected.

As mentioned earlier, it is essential that no one individual controls all of these control points in any hospital system. If one individual controls all these points, the possibility of fraud and abuse is increased. It should be noted that the detection of fraud and abuse is not the intent of external or internal auditing; however, the audit process may uncover one or the other.

PATIENT BUSINESS SERVICES AUDIT INSTRUMENT

Any hospital department or function can be informally audited through the use of an audit survey instrument. The audit instrument should be relatively consistent from one audit period to another. On the other hand, it should also be flexible enough to adjust for the elimination of obsolete functions or systems or for the addition of new functions or systems. In addition, the audit instrument should serve as a reference point from one audit to another so that improvements or weaknesses within the audited area can be tracked.

The audit instrument for the patient business services department shown in Exhibit 13–1 is an example that can be modified for any hospital. It has been designed so that any "no" answer signals the need for further investigation and possible corrective action by management. Answering the questions in this audit instrument, an exception report, is the beginning of the internal audit process. The internal auditor must satisfy himself/herself by observation and testing that the policies, systems, and procedures established by hospital management are, in fact, carried out. After the audit survey has been completed, the internal auditor is responsible for summarizing the findings in a management letter that covers at least the following areas:

- audit approach or methodology used
- findings, including major strengths and weaknesses
- areas in which corrective measures *need* to be taken
- recommendations for improvement
- conclusion

Once the management report has been completed, with appropriate supporting documentation and workpapers, the internal auditor should discuss the report with appropriate members of the hospital's management team.

FLOW CHARTING

Flow charting is probably one of the most useful techniques for documenting and analyzing systems or procedures. The primary purpose of flow charting is to graphically illustrate a complete system. Flow charting has the following advantages over written narratives:[13]

- Standard symbols used in flow charts are generally easier to understand.

Exhibit 13–1 Audit Instrument Form

```
                    Memorial Hospital, Anytown, U.S.A.
                     Patient Business Services Department
                              Audit Instrument
```

	For the Period Ending _____ 19__
Audited by _____	Date _____ 19__

YES	NO	ORGANIZATION
____	____	1. Does the department have an organizational chart?
____	____	2. Does each employee have a job description? If yes, when were the job descriptions last reviewed and updated?
____	____	3. Does each position have established performance standards? If yes, when were the performance standards last reviewed and updated? _____
____	____	4. Is each employee classified in a labor grade and are his/her wages in line with those of similar positions in the rest of the hospital? If yes, when were the labor grades last reviewed and updated? _____
____	____	5. Does the department monitor employee turnover rates for each position? If yes, what is the employee turnover rate for each position?

Position	Annual Turnover Rate
_____	_____
_____	_____
_____	_____

YES	NO	
____	____	6. Are employee production units well defined and capable of being audited? If yes, describe how they are defined and audited:
____	____	7. Does the department conduct inservice education programs? If yes, describe them:
____	____	8. Does the patient account manager report to the chief financial officer? If no, whom does he/she report to:

ACCOUNTING CONTROL

| ____ | ____ | 1. Are all patient accounts receivable subsidiary records reconciled at least monthly? |
| ____ | ____ | 2a. Are all patient accounts receivable records aged at least monthly? |

Exhibit 13–1 continued

YES	NO	
_____	_____	2b. Are they aged by paying agent?
_____	_____	3. Are monthly statements mailed to *all* debtors? If no, why not? _____
		4. Are patient accounts that are written off because of:
_____	_____	a. bad debts
_____	_____	b. courtesy discounts
_____	_____	c. refunds
_____	_____	d. other adjustments
		authorized by appropriate individuals before posting? If yes, who authorizes:
		1. bad debts? _____
		2. courtesy discounts? _____
		3. refunds? _____
		4. other adjustments? (Describe these adjustments) _____
_____	_____	5. Are bad debts adequately monitored after they have been written off? If yes, describe the monitoring process: _____ _____
_____	_____	6. Are all credits to expense recorded and processed through accounts receivable?
_____	_____	a. sales to employees
_____	_____	b. medical record transcriptions
_____	_____	c. sale of obsolete equipment
_____	_____	d. sale of scrap and waste
_____	_____	7. Are patient accounts receivable confirmed by either the internal or external auditor directly and routinely?
_____	_____	8. Are disputed patient accounts receivable reviewed by someone other than an accounts receivable clerk? If yes, who reviews disputed accounts? _____

BUDGETS AND REPORTS

		1. Does the department have:
_____	_____	a. a one-year operating budget?
_____	_____	b. a three-year capital expenditure plan?
_____	_____	2. Are the department's section heads and supervisors involved in the development of these budgets?
_____	_____	3. Does the patient account manager assist in the development of the hospital's cash flow forecast?
_____	_____	4. Is actual performance compared with the department's budgets at least monthly?
		5. Are the following financial statements prepared and reviewed by appropriate members of management every month?
_____	_____	a. Statement of Condition

Exhibit 13-1 continued

YES	NO	
_____	_____	b. Statement of Operations
_____	_____	c. Statement of Financial Changes

COLLECTION ACCOUNTS

YES	NO	
_____	_____	1. Are aged trial balances of agency accounts reviewed monthly?
_____	_____	2. Does the hospital use more than one collection agency?
_____	_____	3. Does the hospital have a written agreement that the agency will return accounts with no payments in six months to the hospital?
_____	_____	4. Are the net agency collection costs computed at least quarterly and compared by agency?

ADMITTING

1. Does the hospital require prepayment for:

YES	NO	
_____	_____	a. inpatient; amount $_____?
_____	_____	b. outpatient; amount $_____?
_____	_____	c. emergency; amount $_____?

2. Does the hospital have separate admitting offices for:

YES	NO	
_____	_____	a. inpatient?
_____	_____	b. outpatient?
_____	_____	c. emergency?

3. Do admitting office personnel report directly to the patient account manager:

YES	NO	
_____	_____	a. inpatient?
_____	_____	b. outpatient?
_____	_____	c. emergency?
_____	_____	4. Does the hospital use patient identification cards?

MAIL RECEIPTS

YES	NO	
_____	_____	1. Are *all* mail receipts opened and listed by someone outside of the patient business services department? If so, who performs these functions?

2. Are copies of the mail receipts listed distributed to the following persons:

YES	NO	
_____	_____	a. chief executive officer?
_____	_____	b. chief financial officer?
_____	_____	c. patient accounts manager?
_____	_____	d. cashier?
_____	_____	3. Are checks immediately stamped "for deposit only"?
_____	_____	4. Does the hospital use a bank lock box for processing mail receipts?

SYSTEMS AND PROCEDURES

YES	NO	
_____	_____	1. Does the department have a manual of standard operating procedures? If yes, when was it last reviewed and updated?

Exhibit 13-1 continued

YES	NO	
___	___	2. Does the department have flow charts of all its major systems and subsystems?
___	___	3. Are completed sample copies of all forms used included in the standard operating procedures manual?
___	___	4. Does the department have a forms control system?

BILLING AND COLLECTION

1. Does the hospital have a written billing and collection policy which includes:
   - ___ ___ a. exact billing schedules?
   - ___ ___ b. criteria for a delinquent account?
   - ___ ___ c. authorized collection actions and procedures?
2. Does the hospital use authorized:
   - ___ ___ a. promissory notes?
   - ___ ___ b. credit cards?
   - ___ ___ c. installment contracts?
3. ___ ___ Are *all* unpaid patient accounts receivable routinely, regularly, and independently mailed to clients?

PATIENT CHARGES

1. ___ ___ Does the department have a published list of all charges set by the hospital?
2. ___ ___ Are department personnel knowledgeable enough to explain to patients how the hospital establishes its charges?
3. ___ ___ Are patient charges checked against patient medical records to assure that *no* charges are lost?
4. ___ ___ Is the rates structure designed to cover all the hospital's financial requirements, including bad debts, allowances, capital, growth, and profit?
5. ___ ___ Are patient charges recorded on a multicharge card to ensure control distribution?
6. ___ ___ Are all patient charges recorded on separate patient account subsidiary ledger files?
7. ___ ___ Are patient charges posted by an individual who does not generate the charges?
8. ___ ___ Are patient charges posted by an individual who does not have responsibility of cash receipts?

CASH PROCESSING

1. ___ ___ Are *all* cash receipts deposited on the day they are received?
2. ___ ___ Are unidentified cash receipts credited to a special account and immediately deposited?
3. ___ ___ Does the hospital have a centralized cashiering system?
4. ___ ___ Does *each* cashier have a separate cash box and imprest fund?
5. ___ ___ Are the cashier's work areas isolated from the hospital personnel?

266 PATIENT ACCOUNT MANAGEMENT

Exhibit 13–1 continued

YES   *NO*

———   ———   6. Do the cashier areas have a "silent alarm" system?
———   ———   7. Does the hospital use a fire-proof safe to store undeposited cash and valuables?
———   ———   8. Are cash receipts recorded by someone other than the individual who receives the cash?

MAIL RETURNS

———   ———   1. Is there an established, written procedure for handling mail returns?
———   ———   2. Have corrective measures been taken to reduce the number of mail returns? If yes, describe these measures:

_____
_____
_____

INSUFFICIENT FUNDS

———   ———   1. Does the hospital have a written policy for handling patient checks that have been returned as "insufficient funds" checks? Describe the policy:

_____
_____
_____

INHOUSE ACCOUNTS

———   ———   1. Do *all* inpatients receive a weekly statement showing the amount they owe while they are still in the hospital? If yes, describe the method used to collect this amount:

_____
_____

———   ———   2. Do representatives of the department visit patients in the hospital to firm up patient payment agreements?
———   ———   3. Does the department use a long-story (30 days or more) report?
———   ———   4. Are third party guarantors billed on an interim basis for accounts that have been classified as "long-stays"?

PETTY CASH

———   ———   1. Does the department use an imprest petty cash fund? If yes, what is the amount ?$_____
———   ———   2. Is only *one* individual responsible for the petty cash fund?
———   ———   3. Does the hospital conduct "spot audits" of the petty cash fund? If yes, how frequently? _____
———   ———   4. Are all petty cash fund disbursements supported by authorized documents and receipts?
———   ———   5. Are *all* cashiers and other personnel responsible for handling cash and valuables bonded?

Exhibit 13–1 continued

YES	NO	
		PATIENT REFUNDS
___	___	1. Are all patient refunds drawn from a separate imprest bank account?
___	___	2. Is each patient refund authorized by an appropriately designated individual? If yes, who authorizes them?
___	___	3. Are the patient refunds documented with a photocopy of the original supporting patient financial statement?
___	___	4. Is the refund bank account reconciled by someone other than the individual who issues or signs checks?

- The chart is necessarily complete because every document in a flow chart must have a point of origin and a point of completion. (Many written narratives are not complete.)

The following narrative description of the requisition and processing of a three-piece patient charge card illustrates this point.

Case Study

The attending physician requisitions a specific pharmaceutical in the patient's medical chart. The attending charge nurse reads the doctor's order and requisitions the drugs via the use of a three-piece pharmacy charge requisition card. The charge card is carried by messenger to the pharmacy. The pharmacist fills the order, prices the cards, and sends the requested drug to the nursing station via messenger. The messenger also returns one portion of the charge card to the nursing station, while the pharmacist keeps one copy and sends a hard copy to the data processing department via messenger. The nurse administers the drug to the patient and confirms this in the nurse's notes in the patient's medical chart. The data processing department posts the charge for the drug on the patient's financial record. After discharge, the patient business services department receives copies of all charges and bills the patient accordingly. The account is stored in the patient accounts receivable file.

This procedure is shown with flow charting symbols in Figure 13–1; the flow chart of the procedure is illustrated in Figure 13–2. This is an example of one of the many methods of flow charting. Two others are the Program Evaluation and Review Technique (PERT) and the Gantt method. They are generally used to plan projects that have many interrelated tasks that

Figure 13-1 Symbols Used for Flow Charting

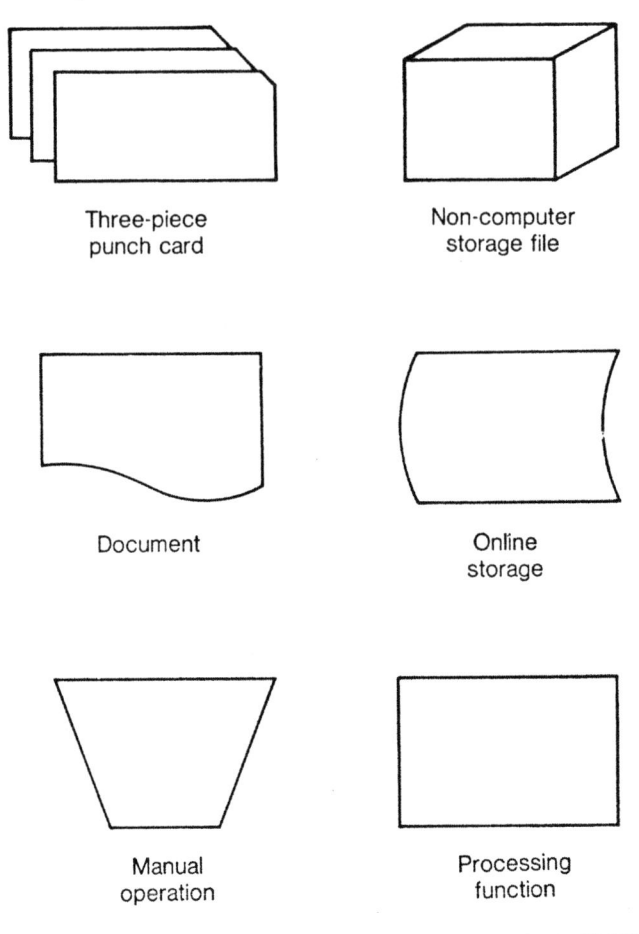

Three-piece punch card	Non-computer storage file
Document	Online storage
Manual operation	Processing function

lead to completion of the project if performed in a given sequence. PERT, also referred to as the Critical Path Method (CPM), is useful in planning and scheduling the sequence of individual tasks and in reviewing the project as a whole.[14]

Although PERT charting uses lines to indicate the flow of work, the length of the lines in no way represents the length of time required to perform interdependent tasks. Therefore, it is difficult for the average user to visualize time relationships in a PERT network diagram. The Gantt chart, named after the person who conceived the idea of plotting tasks instead of time, shows how long a task takes, its earliest starting time (EST), and its latest starting time (LST). Another key difference between

Internal Audit and Control 269

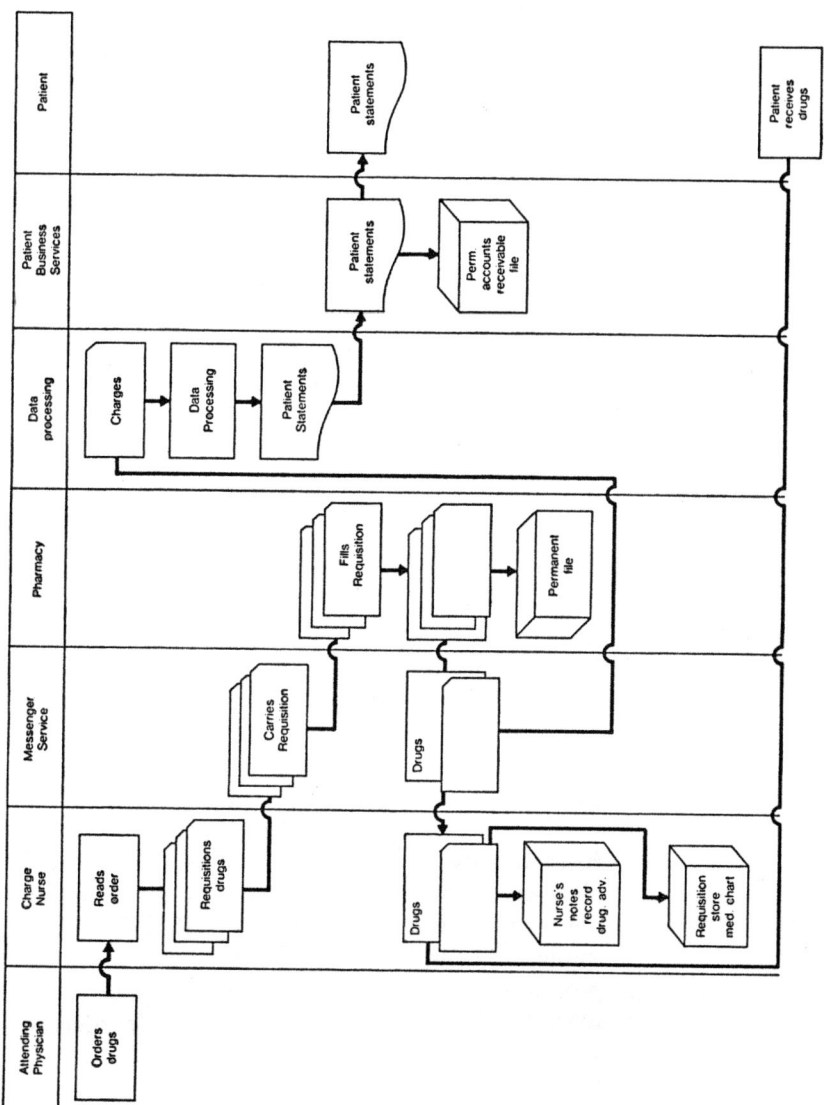

Figure 13-2 Flow Chart of Patient Charges

PERT and Gantt charting is that PERT charting requires the planner to start at the end of the project and work to the start or first task, while Gantt charting requires the planner to start with the first task and identify each task in sequence until the final task is identified. To illustrate the use of these two flow charting methods, assume that the patient account manager wants to implement a hospital courtesy card system to facilitate patient admission and cash collection.

Project: Implement a hospital patient courtesy card system for all inpatients and outpatients of Memorial Hospital, Anytown, U.S.A.

Tasks: The following tasks have been identified as primary components necessary for completion of the project. (Note: The project being illustrated would include more required tasks than are cited in the example, but the number of tasks in the illustrated case has been condensed for ease of understanding.)
1. Locate space for system.
2. Recruit and hire supervisor.
3. Select and order equipment.
4. Prepare site.
5. Install equipment.
6. Recruit and hire support personnel.
7. Train personnel.
8. Develop and conduct publicity campaign.
9. Test system.

Steps:
1. Identify key words in each task to serve as task indicators in charting (see Table 13-1).
2. Estimate how much time will be required to complete each task. (Note: Time can be measured in hours, days, weeks, or months, but time estimates should be consistent throughout the flow charting process.)
3. Identify which tasks must be completed (predecessor) before each task can begin.
4. Start the network at the end of the project by identifying the last event as the end (see Figure 13-3).
5. Plot the predecessor tasks to the final tasks as follows:

Install	5		
Train	7	9	End
Publicity	8		

Table 13–1 PERT Network of Tasks for Implementation of Patient Courtesy Card System, Memorial Hospital, Anytown, U.S.A.

Number	Task Description	Completion Time (Weeks)	Predecessor Tasks
1	Space	1	—
2	Supervisor	4	—
3	Equipment	4	1
4	Preparation	4	3
5	Install	1	4
6	Personnel	4	2
7	Train	2	6
8	Publicity	6	—
9	Final	2	5, 7, 8

6. Plot other tasks as illustrated in Figure 13–3.
7. In order to determine the maximum time required to complete the project, locate the start by dividing the circle in half and placing a zero in the left half as illustrated in Figure 13–4.

$$\text{START} = 0$$

8. Beginning with the start circle, add the time required to complete task number one, and place this number in the left half of the circle for task number one, as follows:

$$1 = 1$$

SPACE   Start: 0 weeks
         Space: 1 week
         Total: 1 week

Continue toward the end circle in this manner, adding the number of weeks required for each task. For example:

$$3 = 5$$

EQUIPMENT   Space: 1 week
             Equipment: 4 weeks
             Total: 5 weeks

272 PATIENT ACCOUNT MANAGEMENT

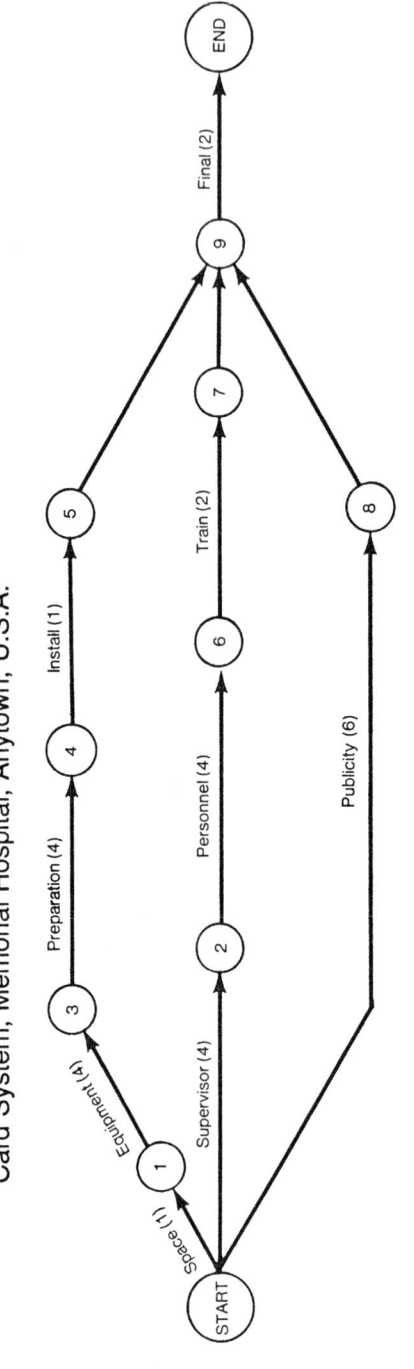

Figure 13–3 PERT Network for Implementation of Patient Courtesy Card System, Memorial Hospital, Anytown, U.S.A.

Figure 13–4 PERT Network for Earliest Starting Times for Patient Courtesy Card System, Memorial Hospital, Anytown, U.S.A.

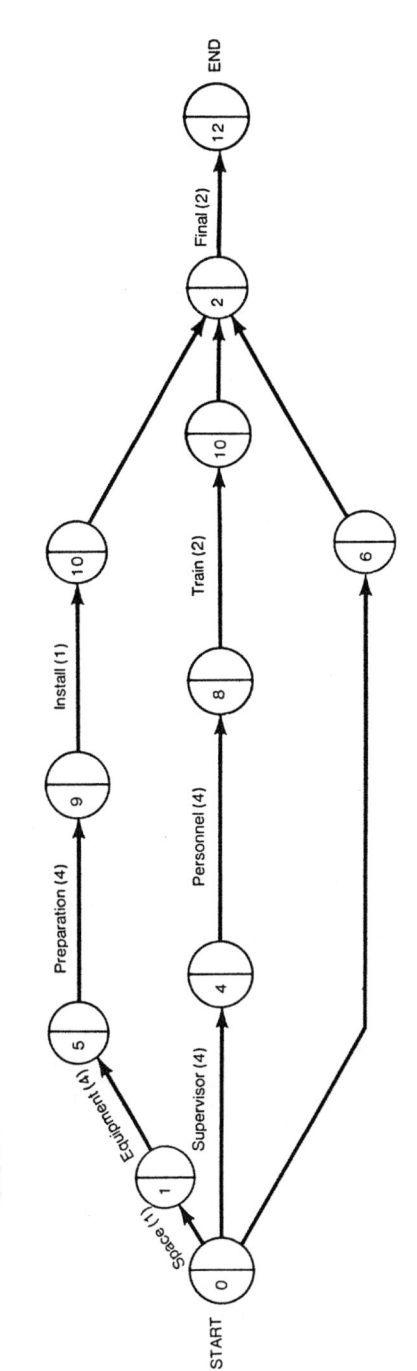

4	=	9
PREPARATION		

Space:	1 week
Equipment:	4 weeks
Preparation:	4 weeks
Total:	9 weeks

5	=	10
INSTALL		

Space:	1 week
Equipment:	4 weeks
Preparation:	4 weeks
Install:	1 week
Total:	10 weeks

Accordingly, the following time schedules are developed for the personnel series of tasks:

Task Number	Description	Time Required	Accumulated Time
2	Hire Supervisor	4 weeks	4 weeks
6	Recruit Personnel	4 weeks	8 weeks
7	Train Personnel	2 weeks	10 weeks

Publicity requires six weeks, indicated in the following manner:

8	=	6
PUBLICITY		

The final testing task requires two weeks; thus at the end, total project time is accumulated as:

END	=	12

Maximum weeks for predecessors is 10 weeks plus 2 weeks, totaling 12 weeks for project.

Figure 13–4 illustrates the EST and shows that 12 weeks is the minimum amount of time for completion of the project. If the LST for the end is 12 weeks, the final task, number 9, must be completed in 10 weeks because completing the final task requires 2 weeks. As shown in Figure 13–5, the EST is placed in the left half of each circle; the LST is placed in the right half of each circle.

The slack time for each task is computed by subtracting the LST from the EST. The critical path is the sequence of tasks with no slack time. An excellent example is the publicity task:

Latest starting time:	4 weeks
Earliest starting time:	0 weeks
Slack time:	4 weeks

There are two critical paths in our example:

Number	Task Description	Weeks	Number	Task Description	Weeks
1	Space	1	2	Supervisor	4
3	Equipment	4	6	Personnel	4
4	Preparation	4	7	Train	2
5	Install	1			
	Total weeks	10		Total weeks	10

Although the PERT flow charting system has proven very effective for professional project planners, it can be fairly described as confusing and difficult to understand for the lay person. Its primary flaw lies in the fact that lines in a PERT chart do not represent the length of time required to complete a given task. Consequently, it is very difficult for one to visualize the relationship of times required to perform the series of tasks that make up the total project.

The Gantt chart, on the other hand, displays the tasks that make up a project in a sequential order and shows the amount of time required to perform each task. In a Gantt chart, the length of the lines corresponds to the amount of time required to complete each task. Figure 13–6 illustrates the way in which a Gantt chart shows these required times.

A Gantt chart is constructed in terms of relevant time frames such as hours, days, weeks, months, or years. In Figure 13–6, weeks have been selected as the relevant time frame for the project. Note that tasks have

276 PATIENT ACCOUNT MANAGEMENT

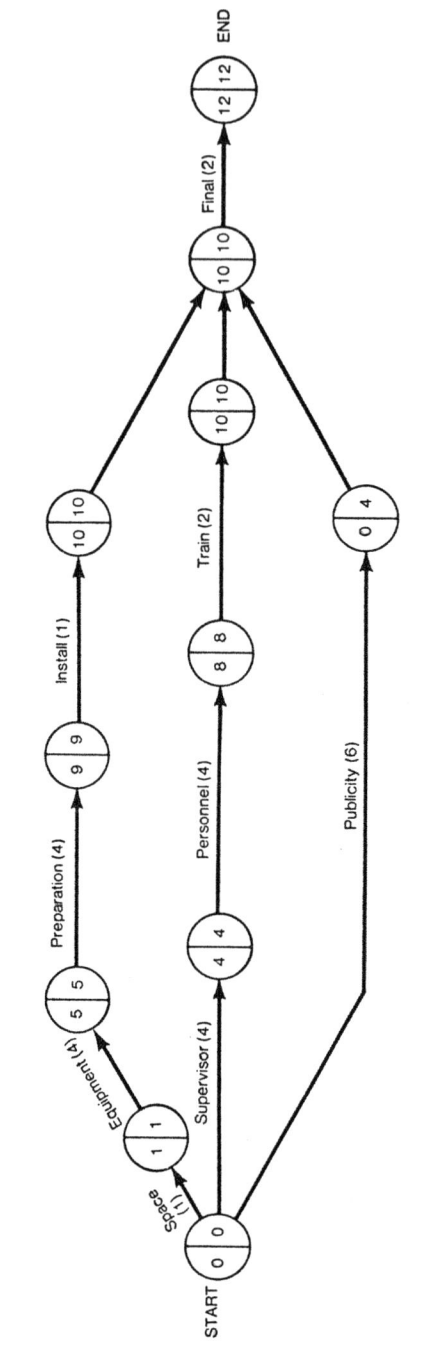

Figure 13–5 PERT Network for Latest Starting Times for Patient Courtesy Card System, Memorial Hospital, Anytown, U.S.A.

Internal Audit and Control 277

Figure 13–6 Gantt Chart for Implementation of Patient Courtesy Card System, Memorial Hospital, Anytown, U.S.A.

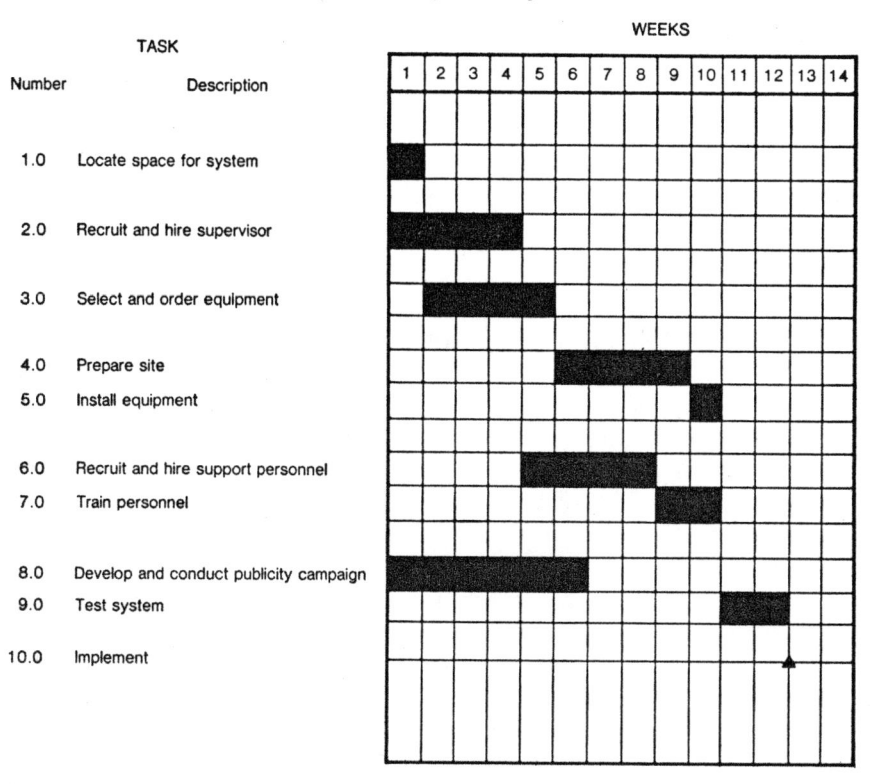

Number	TASK Description	Weeks
1.0	Locate space for system	1
2.0	Recruit and hire supervisor	1–3
3.0	Select and order equipment	2–4
4.0	Prepare site	6–9
5.0	Install equipment	9
6.0	Recruit and hire support personnel	5–9
7.0	Train personnel	9–11
8.0	Develop and conduct publicity campaign	1–7
9.0	Test system	10–12
10.0	Implement	12

been assigned numbers and briefly described. The numbering system used in a Gantt chart should be designed to facilitate identification of subtasks. For example:

- 1.0 Locate space for system.
- 1.1 Determine area required.
- 1.2 Determine utilities required.
- 1.3 Determine most desirable location.
- 1.4 Identify alternative sites.
- 1.5 Review alternatives.
- 1.6 Select site.

Each task, and its subtasks, is listed in the order in which it is most likely to be implemented. On a bar graph, the time required for each task is blocked in, and the position of the block on the chart shows the starting and ending time for the task. After all tasks and subtasks have been listed and plotted on the chart, a solid block triangle is placed on the graph to indicate the project's completion point. If the project planner wants interim checkpoints at specific times, he/she puts an open or white triangle at the places on the graph where checkpoints will occur.

The foregoing discussion of flow charting will acquaint the patient account manager with common techniques used in analyzing existing systems and designing or revising systems. Mastering flow charting techniques can help the patient account manager improve the internal control of patient accounts receivable.

ROLE OF THE PATIENT ACCOUNT MANAGER

As stated in this book's Preface, a silent but steady evolution has taken place in the health care industry in the last decade, particularly in hospitals. The present day patient account manager's position is probably the best example of this silent evolution—more so than any other position in the hospital. The need for a steady and increasing flow of cash into the hospital is critical to its survival today. If a hospital's cash needs are not met, it may well be doomed. Moreover, the patient account manager's role is almost certain to expand and become even more important; the acceleration of change can already be observed.

How the silent evolution will affect the patient account manager depends upon his/her ability to exercise the imagination, drive, and ingenuity needed to cope with the changes that have come and will continue to come. The patient account manager's challenge is to foresee changes and prepare intelligently for them. Certainly, the patient account manager's role is no longer limited to the collection of cash, even though that is a key responsibility of every patient account manager.

NOTES

1. Allen G. Herkimer, Jr., *Concepts in Hospital Financial Management* (Northridge, Calif.: Alfa Associates, Inc., 1973), p. 151.
2. The Institute of Internal Auditors, *Statement of Responsibilities of the Internal Auditor*, May 30, 1957.
3. Ibid.
4. Herkimer, *Concepts in Hospital Financial Management*, pp. 152–153.
5. Ray S. Matylewicz, "Hospital Management and Internal Controls," *Safeguarding the Hospital's Assets* (Oak Brook, Ill.: Hospital Financial Management Association, 1978), p. 3.

6. Charles L. Kampmann, "Internal Control Is for Management," *Safeguarding the Hospital's Assets*, pp. 7–9.
7. Ibid.
8. Ibid.
9. R. Neal Gilbert, "Operational Auditing Checks Effectiveness," *Safeguarding the Hospital's Assets*, p. 176.
10. Ibid.
11. Thomas J. Sullivan, "How the Hospital Can Make Internal Control Work," *Safeguarding the Hospital's Assets*, pp. 43–47.
12 Ibid.
13. Ibid.
14. D. Michael Warner and Don C. Holloway, *Decision Making and Control for Health Administration* (Ann Arbor, Mich.: Health Administration Press, 1978), p. 68.

Index

A

Accounting, 2
  accrual, 30-32
  cash concept of, 30
  fund, 33-34
  general, 27-57
  management, 59-88
  prerequisites of, 34-39
  principles of, 27
  process of, 39-57
  responsibility, 36
Accounting entries, 28
Accounting period, 39
Accounts
  chart of, 34, 35-36, 137, 138
  imprest payroll, 207
Accrual accounting, 30-32
Accuracy degree, 133
Achievement, 118
Acid test (quick) ratio, 225
Activity ratios, 231-233
Actual expenses, 64
Actual performance, 81, 83
Adequate staff of trained personnel, 258
Adjusted standard hours required (ASHR), 113
AHA. *See* American Hospital Association
AHR. *See* Annual Hospital Report

A la carte rates, 190, 191
Algebraic formulas for cost finding, 166
All-inclusive rate, 190, 191
American Hospital Association (AHA), 33, 36, 107, 164, 165, 180
  Chart of Accounts for Hospitals of, 33, 35
American Institute of Certified Public Accountants, 257
Annual accounting period (fiscal year), 39
Annual Hospital Report (AHR), 33, 36, 91-92
Application
  of accounting process, 48-57
  of expense behavior principles, 73-80
Appropriations budget, 125
ASHR. *See* Adjusted standard hours required
Assets, 41, 52, 231, 237
  current, 47, 196, 224
  defensive, 231
  fixed, 232
  net, 41
  net current. *See* Working capital
Attainable cost standard, 134
Attitude of team, 2
Auditing
  external versus internal, 259-260

281

financial versus operational,
    258-259
instruments for, 261, 262-267
internal. See Internal auditing
Authority delegation, 9, 14-15
Average collection period ratio, 238
Average daily revenue uncollected,
    92, 238

B

Bad debt reserve, 252-253
Balance of cash, 196
Balance sheet, 39-41, 52
    comparative, 49, 226-227
    consolidated, 34
Ball, George, 118
Bank float, 196, 197, 200
Basic cost standards, 134
Basic defensive interval, 231
Behavior
    direct variable cost, 157
    expense. See Expense behavior
    step-variable cost, 156
Benefits of standard plans, 25-26
Berman, Howard J., 180
Boedecker, Ray, 15
Borrowings, 197, 200
Break-even analysis ratios, 235
British National Health Service, 181
Budgetary control, 36, 94-98, 117-131
    defined, 117
Budgeted costs, 163
Budgeting Classification Tree, 125,
    126
Budgets, 113, 118, 119, 120
    appropriations, 125
    control. See Control budget
    defined, 117
    direct-variable control, 145-147
    fixed (target), 77, 124, 136, 138,
        139
    flexible. See Variable budget
    functional, 120-124
    moving (rolling), 124

operating, 128, 129, 195
program, 125
project, 125
responsibility, 120-124
rolling (moving), 124
salary, 147-152
target (fixed), 77, 124, 136, 138,
    139
types of, 124-125
variable (flexible). See Variable
    budgets
variances in, 147-152
zero-base, 125

C

California Health Facilities
    Commission, 91
California Hospital Association, 107
CAP. See College of American
    Pathologists
Capital. See Working capital
Capital expenditures, 195, 196, 200
    cash outflows for, 209
    plan for, 129
Carnegie, Andrew, 15
Case studies
    in cost finding, 169-177
    in reimbursement procedures,
        182-189
Cash balance, 196
Cash concept of accounting, 30
Cash disbursements. See Cash
    outflows
Cash flow, 241
    analysis of, 42
    forecast of. See Cash forecasting
    projection of, 43
    statement of, 31, 41-47, 52, 57
Cash forecasting, 44, 119, 120, 129,
    195-217
    methodology in, 201-215
    monitoring of, 215-216
    purpose of, 195-196
    role of patient account manager in,
        215-216

statement of, 198
Cash inflows, 41, 196, 197-199, 201
  See also Revenues
  analysis of, 202, 205
  improving of, 254
  paying agent analysis of, 205
  time lag factor in, 195
Cash management, 195-217
  purpose of, 195-196
Cash outflows, 41-42, 196, 199-200, 201
  See also Costs; Expenses
  analysis of, 201-215
  capital expenditure, 209
  noncapital, 209
  nonsalary. *See* Nonsalary expenses
  prenumbered receipts for, 260
  time lage factor in, 195
Cash receipts. *See* Cash inflows
Cash report form, 216
Cash resource increase, 196
Changes in financial position, 47, 48, 241, 242
"Changes in Working Capital," 47
Charges
  See also Rates
  fixed, 229
  lost, 254
  no, 254
  published. *See* Published rates
  structure of, 2
Chart of accounts, 34, 35-36, 137, 138
Chart of Accounts for Hospitals, AHA, 33, 35
Checks, 260
Collections
  monitoring of, 250-253
  policy on, 22
College of American Pathologists (CAP), 191
Color coding, 23
Command unity, 9, 12
Committed expenses, 70
Communication, 120
  with medical staff, 3

with third-party payers, 3
Comparative balance sheet, 49, 226-227
Comparative statement of operations, 230
Comparisons of cost, 90
Compound accounting entries, 28
Concentration, 119
Condition, statement of. *See* Balance sheet
Connecticut Hospital Association, 107
Consolidated balance sheet, 34
Constant dollars, 69
Contribution, 235
Contribution margin, 235
Control
  budgetary. *See* Budgetary control
  cost, 135
  entry point, 260
  establishment of, 15
  exit point, 260
  internal, 257-258
  processing point, 260
  span of, 9, 12
Control budget, 76, 78, 101
  direct-variable, 145-147
Controllable (direct) operating expenses, 68, 70, 71
Control standard, 81, 83
Cooperation, 120
  with medical staff, 3
Core positions, 95
Cost-benefit analysis, 13
Cost centers, 36
Cost finding, 163-177
  algebraic formulas for, 166
  case study in, 169-177
  defined, 107
  double distribution (double apportionment) method of, 165
  Medicare approach to, 171, 176
  methods of, 165-166
  objectives of, 164
  "Short Formula I" method of, 166
  statistical bases in, 167

stepdown (single apportionment) method of, 165, 176
Costs
See also Expenses
allocation of, 2, 107
analysis of, 70-73
behavior of, 156, 157
budgeted, 163
of carrying patient accounts receivable, 254
classification of, 133, 138
comparisons of, 90
control of, 135
direct variable, 157
economic, 180, 181
historical, 163
operating. *See* Operating expenses
opportunity (lost revenue), 63, 66, 240, 254
out-of-pocket, 179
per production unit, 90, 134
social, 63, 66, 187
standard. *See* Standard costs
of staying in business, 181, 245
step-variable (semi-variable). *See* Step-variable expenses
variability in, 133
variable. *See* Variable expenses
Cost standards, 134
Cost value concept, 38
CPM. *See* Critical Path Method
Credits, 28
Critical path, 275
Critical Path Method (CPM), 268
Current assets, 47, 196, 224
net. *See* Working capital
Current liabilities, 47, 196, 224, 228
Current ratio, 224

D

Daily cash flow analysis form, 42
Daily cash report form, 216
Daily employee self-logging worksheet, 110
Data processing, 3
Debits, 28
Debt ratio, 228
Decision making, 14
Decision packages in zero-base budgeting, 125
Defensive assets, 231
Defensive interval, 231
Degrees of delegation, 14
Delegation
of authority, 9, 14-15
degrees of, 14
guidelines for, 14
mistakes in, 15
of responsibility, 12
Departments
mission of, 3-4
nonrevenue-producing, 165, 167
performance evaluation of, 98-101
productivity per, 90
revenue-producing, 165, 167, 192
structure of, 122, 123
task list for, 109
Deposits from patients, 254
Depreciation, 69, 129, 200, 241
Direct (controllable) expenses, 68, 70, 71
Direct variable control budget, 145-147
Direct variable cost behavior, 157
Disbursement of cash. *See* Cash outflows
Documentation, 7
of financial plan, 118
of proof, 36-38
Dollars, 69
Double distribution (double apportionment) method of cost finding, 165
Double entry-bookkeeping, 28-30
Drucker, Peter F., 69, 89, 90, 119, 180, 181, 245
Duty separation, 257

E

Earliest starting time (EST), 268, 275
Economic costs, 180, 181

Efficiency variance, 80, 81, 152
Elasticity, 65
Employees
　goal-oriented, 120
　incentive plans for, 104-106
　performance evaluation of, 101-104
　productivity per, 90
　self-logging worksheet for, 110
　task-oriented, 120
　time of, 89
Endowment fund, 34
Entry point control, 260
Environment, 4
Equations in cost finding, 166
Equity, 41, 228
EST. *See* Earliest starting time
Estimates, 133
　of expenses, 64
Evaluation of performance. *See*
　Performance evaluation
Execution and implementation, 7, 13
Exit point control, 260
Expenditures. *See* Expenses
Expense behavior principles, 62-69
　application of, 73-80
Expenses
　See also Cash outflows; Costs
　actual, 64
　capital. *See* Capital expenditures
　committed, 70
　depreciation, 69, 129, 200, 241
　direct (controllable), 70, 71
　estimated, 64
　fixed, 64, 70, 76, 133, 137, 145
　inflation, 69
　nonsalary. *See* Nonsalary expenses
　operating. *See* Operating expenses
　opportunity. *See* Opportunity costs
　planned, 64
　programmed, 70, 199, 209
　replacement, 69, 70
　salary and payroll, 69
　social. *See* Social costs
　step-variable, 64, 65, 157
　variable. *See* Variable expenses
　variances in, 84, 152-157

External auditing versus internal
　auditing, 259-260
External environment, 4
External reporting, 59

F

Fact finding, 14
*Factors to Evaluate in the
　Establishment of Hospital Charges,*
　180
Feedback, 15, 129
Financial analysis, 219-243
Financial auditing versus operational
　auditing, 258-259
Financial plan. *See* Budget
Financial position statement. *See*
　Balance sheet
Financial ratios, 219-222
　types of, 222-237
Financial requirements, 180-181
Financial statements, 39, 241-243
Fiscal year (annual accounting
　period), 39
Fixed asset turnover, 232
Fixed budget (target budget), 77,
　124, 136, 138, 139
Fixed charges ratio, 229, 231
Fixed expenses, 64, 70, 76, 133, 137,
　145
Fixed period budgets, 124
Fixed positions, 95
Flexible budgets. *See* Variable
　budgets
Flow charts, 23, 24, 261-278
Forecasting
　cash. *See* Cash forecasting
　judgment in, 133
　statistical, 128
Formalization, 7
Format of job description, 17
Forms
　audit instrument, 262-267
　daily cash flow analysis, 42
　daily cash report, 216

standard, 23
Formulas in cost finding, 166
Freedom, 118
Functional budgeting, 120-124
Functional cost center, 36
Fund accounting, 33-34
Fund-raising drives, 199
Funds
   endowment, 34
   operating, 34
   plant replacement and expansion, 34
   restricted, 33, 34
   specific purpose, 34
   unrestricted, 33, 34

G

Gantt charts, 267, 270, 275, 277
General accounting, 27-57
General ledger, 39
Goal-oriented employees, 120
Goals, 12, 118, 120, 128
   See also Mission; Objectives; Purpose
Groner, Patrick N., 106
Guidelines for delegation, 14

H

HCFA. *See* Health Care Financing Administration
Health Care Financing Administration (HCFA), 33, 36
Health and Human Services (HHS), 36
   Annual Hospital Report (AHR) of, 33, 36, 91-92
HHS. *See* Health and Human Services
Historical costs, 163
Horngren, Charles T., 59, 134
Humantology, 120

I

IBM. *See* International Business Machines
Identification
   of primary responsibility centers, 9
   of resources, 13
Implementation and execution, 7, 13
Imprest payroll account, 207
Improving of cash inflow, 254
Incentive plans of employees, 104-106
Income and expense statement. *See* Statement of operations
Income statement. *See* Statement of operations
Increase in cash resources, 196
Indirect (uncontrollable) operating expenses, 68
Inflation expense, 69
Inflows. *See* Cash inflows
Initial documentation, 7
Inputs (employee time), 89
   See also Production units; Productivity
Interest charges on outstanding patient accounts, 254
Internal auditing
   defined, 256-257
   element of surprise in, 256
   versus external auditing, 259-260
   and organizational chart, 256
Internal control, 257-258
   defined, 257
Internal reporting, 59
International Business Machines (IBM), 15
Inventory turnover, 232
Investments, 197, 200
Involvement approach to production standard development, 108

J

JCAH. *See* Joint Commission on Accreditation of Hospitals

Job analysis, 15-16
Job description, 16-17, 18
  format of, 17
  performance standards in, 94
Joint Commission on Accreditation of Hospitals (JCAH), 196
Journals, 38-39
Judgment in forecasting, 133

K

Kampmann, Charles L., 257

L

Latest starting time (LST), 268, 275
Leadership role of patient account manager, 120
Ledgers, 38-39
  general, 39
Leverage ratios, 228-231
Liabilities, 41, 52
  current, 47, 196, 224, 228
Liquidity of patient accounts receivable, 237-241
Liquidity ratios, 224-227
Lost charges, 254
Lost revenue (opportunity costs), 63, 66, 240, 254
LST. *See* Latest starting time

M

Macro production units, 91-92, 167
Macro service units, 191
Management
  cash, 195-217
  defined, 1
  history of, 90
  for results, 118
  theories of, 2, 12
Management accounting, 59-88

Management planning
  defined, 6
  operational, 12
  steps in, 8
Management reporting, 60-62
Management style, 2, 117, 130
Managing in Turbulent Times, 245
Margin
  contribution, 235
  profit, 234
Market analysis, 249
Market segmentation, 249
Matrix of segmentation, 250
Maximum efficiency cost standard, 134
McGregor, Douglas, 2
Measurement
  motion time, 108
  standard unit of, 91
  of work. *See* Production units
Medical records, 3
Medical staff cooperation, 3
Medicare
  and cost finding, 171, 176
  reporting system under, 33
Medicare-Medicaid Antifraud and Abuse Amendments (PL 95-142), 36
Methods, 25
Micro production units, 92, 167, 169
Micro service units, 191
Mission, 128
  See also Goals; Objectives; Purpose
  defined, 4-6
  departmental, 3-4
Mistakes in delegating, 15
Monitoring
  of accounts in collection, 250-253
  of cash forecast, 215-216
Motion time measurement (MTM), 108
Moving (rolling) budgets, 124
MTM. *See* Motion time measurement
Multilateral approach, 12, 13, 118

N

Narration form of written procedures, 23
Negative elasticity, 65
Nesbitt, W. H., 14
Net assets, 41
Net current assets. *See* Working capital
Net operating profits, 241
Net worth, 52
    ratio of patient accounts receivable to, 240
No charges, 254
Noncapital cash outflows, 209
Nonrevenue-producing departments, 165, 167
Nonsalary expenses, 69, 137, 208
    programmed, 199
    variable, 154-155, 199
    variances in, 84, 152-157
Normal task time, 112
    per production unit, 108

O

Objectives, 5, 12, 118, 120, 128
    See also Goals; Mission; Purpose
    of cost control program, 135
    of cost finding, 164
    setting of, 12, 13
Open communication with third party reimbursement agencies, 3
Operating budget, 128, 129, 195
Operating cash balance, 196
Operating expenses, 63, 66, 68, 69, 181, 245
    direct (controllable), 68
    indirect (uncontrollable), 68
Operating funds, 34
Operating profits, 241
Operating revenues, 196
Operational auditing versus financial auditing, 258-259
Operational management planning process steps, 12
Operations statement. *See* Statement of operations
Opportunity costs (lost revenue), 63, 66, 240, 254
Optimum number of subordinates per supervisor, 9
Organization, 7
Organizational chart, 34, 35, 37
    internal auditor's position in, 256
Organizational structure, 6-14, 257
    chart of. *See* Organizational chart
    patient business services department, 123
    planning process for, 7
    PSR, 4, 9, 11, 16, 122
    rules of, 9
    as standard plan, 21
    traditional, 4, 10
Outflows. *See* Cash outflows
Out-of-pocket costs, 179
Outputs, 89, 133
    units of. *See* Production units
Outstanding patient accounts, 254

P

Patient deposits, 254
Patient service representative (PSR), 4, 9, 11, 16, 122
Payer classification, 248
Paying agent cash inflow analysis, 205
Payment, 248-249
    See also Reimbursement
    prospective, 163, 248
    versus published charge, 247
    retrospective, 164, 248
    schedules of, 203
Payroll account, 207
Performance
    actual, 81, 83
    departmental, 98-101

evaluation of. *See* Performance
evaluation
standards of. *See* Performance
standards
Performance evaluation, 5, 7, 13, 14,
89, 98, 129
employee, 101-104
Performance factor, 113
calculation worksheet for, 114
Performance standards, 3, 13, 94, 96,
103, 105, 106, 118
development of, 108-116
involvement approach to, 108
in job description, 94
predetermined, 108
variable approach to, 98
Personal, fatigue and delay (PFD)
factor, 108, 109, 111, 112
PERT. *See* Program Evaluation and
Review Technique
PFD. *See* Personal, fatigue, and
delay
PL 92-603 Social Security
Amendments, 248
PL 95-142 (Medicare-Medicaid
Antifraud and Abuse
Amendments), 36
Planned expenses, 64
Planning
management. *See* Management
planning
organizational structure, 7
standard, 21-26
Plant replacement and expansion
fund, 34
Policies, 21-22
collection, 22
defined, 21
sound, 258
Pope, Alexander, 255
Positions
See also Staff
core, 95
fixed, 95
variable, 96, 97
Positive elasticity, 65

Predetermined production standard
approach, 108
Prenumbered cash receipts, 260
Prenumbered checks, 260
Prepayment for service, 254
Prerequisites of accounting systems,
34-39
Preview, 7
Primary responsibility center
identification, 9
Principles of accounting, 27
Principles of expense behavior,
62-69, 73-80
Procedures, 22-25
defined, 23
reimbursement, 182-189
sound, 258
written, 23
Processing point control, 260
Production
defined, 13
standards of. *See* Performance
standards
trend chart on, 115
units of. *See* Production units
Production units, 89, 90-92, 101, 103,
106, 107, 119, 138, 139, 167
cost per, 90, 134
macro, 91-92, 167
micro, 92, 167, 169
normal task time per, 108
selection of, 92-94
standard time for, 111, 112
Productivity
defined, 89
improvement program for, 89-116
per employee and/or department,
90
Profit, 180, 245
operating, 241
Profitability ratios, 233-235
Profit and loss statement. *See*
Statement of operations
Profit margin ratio, 234
Profit planning ratios, 235-237
Program budget, 125

Program Evaluation and Review
  Technique (PERT), 267, 268, 270,
  271, 272, 273, 275, 276
Programmed expenses, 70, 199, 209
Project budget, 125
Projection of cash flow, 43
Proof documentation, 36-38
Prospective payment systems, 163,
  248
Provider Reimbursement Review
  Board (PRRB), 177
PRRB. See Provider Reimbursement
  Review Board
PSR. See Patient service
  representative
Published rates
  versus payment, 247
  third party impact on, 181-182
Purpose
  See also Goals; Mission; Objectives
  of cash forecasting, 195-196
  of cash management, 195-196
  statement of, 128

Q

Quick ratio (acid test ratio), 225

R

Rate of turnover, 231, 238
Rates
  See also Charges
  a la carte, 190, 191
  all-inclusive, 190, 191
  published. See Published rates
  setting of. See Rate setting
  standard. See Standard rates
  variance in, 80, 81, 83, 152, 153
Rate setting, 163, 190-194
  prospective, 163, 248
Ratio analysis of patient accounts
  receivable, 50-52

Ratios
  activity, 231-233
  average collection period, 238
  break-even analysis, 235
  current, 224
  debt, 228
  financial, 219-237
  fixed charges, 229, 231
  leverage, 228-231
  liquidity, 224-227
  profitability, 233-235
  profit margin, 234
  profit planning, 235-237
  quick (acid test ratio), 225
  receivables to charges, 239
  receivables to net worth, 240
  return on net worth or equity, 234
  times interest earned, 229, 231
Receivables-to-charges ratio, 239
Receivables-to-net-worth ratio, 240
Receivables turnover, 233
Reimbursement
  See also Payment
  case study of, 182-189
  third-party. See Third-party payers
Relative value units (RVU), 191
Relevant range of activity (RRA)
  method of staffing, 98
Replacement expense, 69, 70
Reporting
  daily cash, 216
  external, 59
  internal, 59
  management, 60-62
  Medicare, 33
Reserve for bad debts, 252-253
Resources
  cash, 196
  identification of, 13
Responsibility accounting, 36
Responsibility budgeting, 120-124
Responsibility centers, 9
Responsibility delegation, 12
Restricted funds, 33, 34
Retrospective payment systems, 164,
  248

Return on net worth or equity ratio, 234
Revenue and expense statement. *See* Statement of operations
Revenue-producing centers, 165, 167, 192
Revenues
See also Cash inflows
lost (opportunity costs), 63, 66, 240, 254
operating, 196
Review. *See* Evaluation
Reward level in employee incentive plans, 106
Role of patient account manager, 1, 120, 278
in cash forecasting, 215-216
leadership, 120
Rolling (moving) budgets, 124
RRA. *See* Relevant range of activity
Rules of organizational design, 9
RVU. *See* Relative value units

S

Salary variance, 82
analysis of, 80, 147-152
Schedules of payment, 203
Seawell, L. Vann, 27, 38, 180
Segmentation of patient accounts receivable, 249-250
Self-evaluation, 7
Self-logging employee involvement method, 113
Self-pay, 248
Semi-variable cost. *See* Step-variable costs
Separation of duties, 257
Service units, 191
Sherman, Harvey, 14
"Short Formula 1" method of cost finding, 166
Simultaneous equations, 166
Single accounting entries, 28

Single apportionment (stepdown) method of cost-finding, 165, 176
Social costs, 63, 66, 187
Social Security Amendments in Public Law 92-603, 248
Social services, 3
Sound policies and procedures, 258
Span of control, 9, 12
Specific purpose fund, 34
Staff, 94-98
See also Positions
adequate, 258
elasticity factor in, 157
requirement for, 96, 97, 98
RRA method of, 98
step-variable, 157-161
variable requirement for, 96, 97
volume-range method of determination of requirement for, 98
Standard costs
defined, 136
development of, 135-136
and variable bugeting, 134-135
Standard forms, 23
Standard methods, 25
Standard performance, 106
Standard plans, 21-26
benefits of, 25-26
organizational structures as, 21
Standard production unit time, 111, 112
Standard rates, 74, 98, 101
defined, 136
development of, 135-136
Standards
control, 81, 83
cost, 134
of performance. *See* Performance standards
of production. *See* Performance standards
Standard time development worksheet, 111, 112
Standard unit of measurement (SUM), 91

Statement of operations, 45, 46, 52, 56, 223, 230, 241
  comparative, 230
Statements
  cash flow, 31, 41-47, 52, 57
  cash forecast, 198
  of changes in financial position, 47, 48, 241, 242
  of condition. *See* Balance sheet
  financial, 39, 241-243
  of financial position. *See* Balance sheet
  income and expense. *See* Statement of operations
  profit and loss. *See* Statement of operations
  of purpose, 128
  of sources and application of funds. *See* Statement of changes in financial position
Statistical bases in cost finding, 167
Statistical forecast, 128
Staying-in-business costs, 181, 245
Stepdown (single apportionment) method of cost finding, 165, 176
Step-by-step narration form of written procedures, 23
Step-variable (semi-variable) expenses, 64, 65, 133, 157
  behavior of, 156
Step-variable staffing, 157-161
Style of management, 2, 117, 130
Subordinate number per supervisor, 9
SUM. *See* Standard unit of measurement
Surprise element in internal audits, 256

T

Target (fixed) budget, 77, 134, 136, 138, 139
Target level in employee incentive plans, 105
Target production level (TPL), 113
Task frequency mix factors, 109
Task list for department, 109
Task-oriented employees, 120
Task time, 108, 112
Team, 14, 15, 118
  attitude of, 2
Theory X, 2, 12
Theory Y, 2, 12
Theory Z, 2, 12
Third-party payers, 248
  open communication with, 3
  and published rates, 181-182
  and retrospective payments, 164, 248
Time development worksheets, 111, 112
Time lag factors, 195, 201, 203, 208
  cash inflow, 195
  cash outflow, 195
Times interest earned ratio, 229, 231
Total asset turnover ratio, 233
TPL. *See* Target production level
Traditional organizational structure, 4, 9, 10
Traditional patient business services department structure, 122, 123
Turnover
  accounts receivable, 231, 233, 238
  asset, 231, 232
  inventory, 232
  rate of, 231, 238

U

Uncontrollable (indirect) operating expenses, 68
Unilateral approach, 12, 13, 118
Units
  of measurement, 91
  of output. *See* Production units
  of production. *See* Production units
  relative value, 191
  of service, 191

Unity of command, 9, 12
Unrestricted funds, 33, 34
Usage variance, 153

V

Variable approach to production
   standards, 98
Variable budget (flexible budget), 73,
   124
   development of, 136-144
   purpose of, 133-134
   and standard costs, 134-135
   worksheet for, 140-141
Variable expense budget, 76
Variable expenses, 64, 65, 71, 72, 74,
   76, 133, 209, 210
   behavior of, 157
   direct, 157
   nonsalary, 154-155, 199
Variable staffing requirement, 96, 97
Variance analysis, 80-87
   salary, 80
   and step-variable staffing, 157-161
Variances
   budget, 147-152
   efficiency, 80, 81, 152
   nonsalary expense, 84, 152-157
   rate, 80, 81, 83, 152, 153

salary, 82
usage, 153
work volume, 83
Volume-range method of staffing
   requirement determination, 98
Volume of work, 133
   variances in, 83

W

Washington State Hospital
   Commission, 187
Weeks, Lewis E., 180
Weighted average monthly cash
   inflow percentage method, 203
Westinghouse Electric Corporation,
   14
Work
   measurement of. *See* Production
      units
   volume of. *See* Volume of work
Working capital, 47-48
   defined, 47
Written procedures, 23

Z

Zero-base budgeting, 125

About the Author

ALLEN G. HERKIMER, JR., entered the hospital industry in 1957 as a business office manager (patient account manager) of a small Connecticut hospital. Mr. Herkimer is presently an Assistant Professor in the Department of Health Science, California State University, Northridge, and Adjunct Professor at the University of Southern California. He is a faculty member of the Western Network for Education in Health Administration affiliated with the University of California at Berkeley and a member of the Graduate Programs Coordinating Committee of the Healthcare Financial Management Education Foundation, sponsored by the W.K. Kellogg Foundation. He is also a principal of Alfa Management Services, a healthcare consulting firm, headquartered in Northridge, California.

Before entering the academic field, Mr. Herkimer had over 20 years of experience within the nontaxable and taxable segments of the hospital industry, including service as president of a rural medical service corporation, vice-president of a health care management company, principal of a national consulting firm, as well as hospital controller.

From 1969 through 1972, he was Project Director of the nation's first Incentive Reimbursement Experiment funded by the Social Security Administration and Connecticut Blue Cross, and he served as Co-Chairman of the President's Cost of Living Council, National Commission on Productivity's Panel on Hospital Financial Management. In 1974, he created and directed the Hospital Resource Unit (HRU) Project. The objective on this project was to develop a quantitative measure of health care services.

He has authored numerous trade journal articles and published two books. His most recent book, *Understanding Hospital Financial Management,* published by Aspen Systems Corporation, was selected by the American Journal of Nursing as its Book-of-the-Year in 1979.

Mr. Herkimer is a Fellow, National Life Member Certified Patient Account Manager, and past National Director of the Healthcare Financial Management Association and, in 1975, received the Association's Frederick C. Morgan Award given to an individual who has made an outstanding contribution to the field of health care financial management. In addition, he is a member of the Hospital Management Systems Society, National Life Member of American Guild of Patient Account Managers, and member of the American College of Hospital Administrators. He received his Bachelor of Science degree from Syracuse University and his Master of Business Administration degree from the University of Bridgeport, Connecticut. Currently, he is a doctoral candidate at the University of La Verne's School of Management.